INSTRUCTOR'S MANUAL

for

THE NEW LEADERSHIP CHALLENGE:

CREATING A FUTURE

FOR NURSING

Sheila C. Grossman, Ph.D. APRN
Associate Professor and Director, Undergraduate Program
Fairfield University
Fairfield, CT 06430-5195

F. A. DAVIS COMPANY • PHILADELPHIA

F. A. Davis Company
1915 Arch Street
Philadelphia, PA 19103

Printed in the United States of America

Last digit indicated print number 10 9 8 7 6 5 4 3 2

Managing Publisher, Nursing: Lisa A. Biello
Acquisitions Editor: Joanne P. DaCunha, RN, MSN
Production Editor: Michael Schnee
Cover Designer: Louis J. Forgione

ISBN
0-8036-0596

TABLE OF CONTENTS

PREFACE

This manual assists the instructor in using *The New Leadership Challenge: Creating a Preferred Future for Nursing* to teach nursing leadership and facilitate the development of nurses and student nurses as leaders. The text can be used in a senior-level "Nursing Leadership and Management" course, in a graduate course in leadership, or throughout a program with an integrated curriculum. Because preparation for a leadership role begins at the undergraduate level and continues throughout one's career, this book also may be used in staff development or continuing education leadership workshops for nurses who want to increase their leadership ability. This manual is designed to help instructors reinforce the concept that all nurses — not just those who are in positions of authority (e.g., directors, supervisors, and managers) — need to develop their leadership abilities and help create nursing's preferred future.

Nurses who are leaders need to reflect self-reliance, a positive self-image, self awareness, determination, effective group skills, critical thinking ability, perseverance, patience, responsibility, accountability, optimism, high expectations, energy, courage, strength, adaptability, and enthusiasm. It is necessary, therefore, to identify strategies that can help learners to acquire or further develop such leadership skills as risk taking, conflict management, managing change, goal setting, flexibility, assertiveness, team building, persuasion, communication, collaboration, mentoring, and networking. This manual helps identify such strategies.

This manual also addresses how some of the more "traditional" management techniques (e.g., planning, decision making, time management, delegation, use of authority and power, change, staffing, quality improvement, financial management, and risk management) can be used to enhance learning about leadership. Although all managers are not necessarily leaders, those who are skilled at management may be well on their way to being skilled at leadership. Thus, some attention to management development can enhance leadership development. This manual is designed to help bridge the gap between nurses' knowledge about management and how that knowledge can help them be effective leaders.

Teaching Strategies

The accompanying text lays a solid foundation for understanding leadership. This manual suggests how the instructor can build on the basis provided in the text to develop class sessions and design learning activities that enhance student understanding. Samples of overheads (in addition to those that could be made by copying and magnifying tables and figures in the text itself) and step-by-step learning activities are provided to assist the instructor in facilitating the students'/nurses' accomplishment of each chapter's objectives.

It is expected that while some review of basic content may be needed during class sessions, most class sessions will be similar to seminars, and the activities provided here could be used to stimulate discussion. Some of the text's critical thinking exercises can also be used as "jumping-off points" to initiate discussion of the topics at hand. Maximum participation from all students might be enhanced if class participation were evaluated and graded; therefore, Appendix A is provided to offer one approach to grading class participation.

Evaluation

Given the nature of leadership and the integrative nature of the concept, it would seem that essay-like questions and action projects may be more appropriate for evaluating students' ability to integrate and apply theory and their understanding of this complex concept. Instructors might consider using midterm and final exams, graded class participation that reflects a significant portion of the course grade (e.g., 15%–20%), and a written and/or oral presentation of a leadership project. Appendix B offers one example of guidelines to and evaluation of a leader analysis paper.

Annotated Bibliography

Appendix C is another source of assistance for the teacher of leadership. It offers annotated bibliographies of several of the classic, unique, or significant texts in the leadership field. It is the author's hope that these annotations will help the teacher facilitate dynamic discussions with students on various aspects of leadership.

THE NATURE OF LEADERSHIP... DISTINGUISHING LEADERSHIP FROM MANGEMENT

1

INTRODUCTION

Leaders do the right thing" and "mangers do things right" are two statements that seem to represent the prevailing idea of the difference between a leader and a manager. Actually, both statements apply to leaders, and it is the main goal of this chapter to facilitate students' understanding of this point. It is also imperative to convey to learners that ordinary people can do extraordinary things if they use their leadership ability. Also of significance is the understanding that all nurses can and must be leaders; we (1987) describe five action of leaders that demonstrate how ordinary people who are not in authority positions can be effective in leadership.

- ◆ Challenge the process by searching for growth

- ◆ Motivate others to work together and plan for the future

- ◆ Facilitate others to work together

- ◆ Be a role model for others

- ◆ Give recognition to the accompiishments of others

OBJECTIVES

- ◆ Compare and contrast the major theories of leadership.

- ◆ Discuss the essential elements of leadership.

- ◆ Describe the nine "tasks of leadership."

- ◆ Distinguish leadership from management.

- ◆ Create a personal definition of leadership that reflects its essential elements.

KEY WORDS

Authority	Leadership Styles	Preceptin	Vision
Change	Management	Risk-Taking	
Communication	Mentoring	Role Modeling	
Leadership	Power	Stewardship	

ACTIVITIES

1. Have the students practice leadership by being a committee chair, co-chair, or officer in the Student Nurses Association (SNA); a Sigma Theta Tau chapter A School of Nursing committee; or a community, church, or university group. Emphasize the significance of developing one's leadership skills by identifying opportunities to practice leadership and participating fully as an officer or chairperson. Students should keep journals that describe their participation at each meeting and analyze their strengths and weaknesses in leading the group and the strengths and limitations of various group members. Instructors should evaluate each entry in a timely manner after each meeting in order to give students constructive feedback on their leadership practices. At the end of the semester, students should submit a comprehensive report that documents the meetings (e.g., dates, names of participants, brief description of activities and goals accomplished, plans for future meetings), as well as a summary of how they would lead differently if they were given another opportunity.

2. Have the students complete the Least-Preferred Coworker (LPC) Scale (Fiedler, Chemers, and Mahar, 1976) (Figure 1–1) to determine their leadership style. Have them discuss how different situations would require specific leadership styles. Next, have the students complete the Leadership Style Test (Douglas, 1992) (Figure 1–2) to assess the type of style they prefer when relating to subordinates. (Note that this test uses the term "subordinates," not "followers"; discuss this point with students.) The purpose of these exercises is to promote growth in students' roles as leaders in their selected committee settings (see Activity #1) and in other situations.

3. Because leadership has at least 350 different definitions, none of which gives the best definition of the concept, the exact meaning of the term is open to discussion and analysis. Have all students write their personal definition of leadership during the first class session. Then, during the final class session, have students write a second definition. At this point, return the original definitions and ask the students to evaluate their effectiveness in practicing leadership after being on a committee (see Activity #1) and (b) comparing it with Gardner's (1989) nine tasks of leadership and determining how many of Gardner's tasks they incorporated into their final definition. Students should share their ideas in small groups so that everyone gets the opportunity to discuss his or her growth.

4. Use Text Table 1.1, "Differences between Leadership and Management," to trigger a discussion on the similarities and differences between leadership and management. Examine each of the elements presented: position, power base, goals/visions, innovative ideas, risk level, degree of order, nature of activities, focus, perspective, degree of "freedom." And markers, and tell them to draw their depiction of leadership and management. After students have shared their drawings and interpreted them to the class, share your own depiction of the two concepts. The students could also analyze leadership and management activities in a more concrete fashion by identifying which of their nurse managers' activities demonstrate leadership and which constitute management.

5. Have the students write a paper analyzing and comparing a nurse and a non-nurse leader or multiple leaders. Appendix B provides examples of how this assignment could be designed and graded. Such an assignment could take the place of other activities suggested here or in Chapter 1 of the text because it incorporates so many objectives for this area of study.

REFERENCES

Douglas, L. M. 1992. *The effective nurse leader and manager.* 4th ed, 25–28. St. Louis: Mosby.

Fiedler, F., M. Chemers, and L. Mahar. 1976. *Improving leadership effectiveness: the leader match concept.* New York: J Wiley.

Gardner, J. 1989. The tasks of leadership. In *Contemporary issues in leadership.* 2d ed, 24–33. Edited by W. E. Rosenbach and R. Taylor. Boulder, CO: Westview Press.

Kouzes, J., and B. Posner. 1987. *The leadership challenge.* San Francisco: Jossey-Bass

Figure 1–1

LEAST-PREFERRED COWORKER (LPC) SCALE

(Fiedler, Chemers, and Mahar 1976)

Most people are effective leaders in one situation and not in another, depending on their leadership style and the leadership situation. Here is a simple test, developed by Fiedler, Chemers, and Mahar (1976), to determine your leadership style. Fiedler and colleagues found that people's leadership styles are reflected in their LPC ratings, or the way that they view their *least-preferred coworker*. In jobs you have done throughout your career, some coworkers have been easier to work with than others. Consider the person you had or have the most problems working with and rate that person according to the 18 characteristics below. After you have taken the test, add up the numbers under each "X" that you marked and record that number in the column on the right. Remember that there are no right or wrong answers. Each type of leader is best suited for a particular leadership situation. Now, rate your leadership style.

Pleasant	__ __ __ __ __ __ __ __	Unpleasant	_____
	8 7 6 5 4 3 2 1		
Friendly	__ __ __ __ __ __ __ __	Unfriendly	_____
	8 7 6 5 4 3 2 1		
Rejecting	__ __ __ __ __ __ __ __	Accepting	_____
	1 2 3 4 5 6 7 8		
Tense	__ __ __ __ __ __ __ __	Relaxed	_____
	1 2 3 4 5 6 7 8		
Distant	__ __ __ __ __ __ __ __	Close	_____
	1 2 3 4 5 6 7 8		
Cold	__ __ __ __ __ __ __ __	Warm	_____
	1 2 3 4 5 6 7 8		
Supportive	__ __ __ __ __ __ __ __	Hostile	_____
	8 7 6 5 4 3 2 1		
Boring	__ __ __ __ __ __ __ __	Interesting	_____
	1 2 3 4 5 6 7 8		

4

Quarrelsome	_____	_____	_____	_____	_____	_____	_____	_____	Harmonious	_____
	1	2	3	4	5	6	7	8		
Gloomy	_____	_____	_____	_____	_____	_____	_____	_____	Cheerful	_____
	1	2	3	4	5	6	7	8		
Open	_____	_____	_____	_____	_____	_____	_____	_____	Guarded	_____
	8	7	6	5	4	3	2	1		
Backbiting	_____	_____	_____	_____	_____	_____	_____	_____	Loyal	_____
	1	2	3	4	5	6	7	8		
Untrustworthy	_____	_____	_____	_____	_____	_____	_____	_____	Trustworthy	_____
	1	2	3	4	5	6	7	8		
Considerate	_____	_____	_____	_____	_____	_____	_____	_____	Inconsiderate	_____
	8	7	6	5	4	3	2	1		
Nasty	_____	_____	_____	_____	_____	_____	_____	_____	Nice	_____
	1	2	3	4	5	6	7	8		
Agreeable	_____	_____	_____	_____	_____	_____	_____	_____	Disagreeable	_____
	8	7	6	5	4	3	2	1		
Insincere	_____	_____	_____	_____	_____	_____	_____	_____	Sincere	_____
	1	2	3	4	5	6	7	8		
Kind	_____	_____	_____	_____	_____	_____	_____	_____	Unkind	_____
	8	7	6	5	4	3	2	1		

Total all numbers in the right-hand column to arrive at your LPC score and determine what kind of leader you are. The leader match concept identifies leaders as "task-motivated" or "relationship-motivated."

If you are a **high LPC leader** (if you scored 64 or higher), you are relationship-motivated. You are more concerned with personal relations, more sensitive to the feelings of others, and better at heading off conflict than a task-motivated leader. You use good relations with individuals in your association to get the job done. You prefer situations in which you have a moderate amount of control because you can use group relations to ease anxiety and tension and to reduce conflict. You are patient, considerate, and concerned with the feelings and opinions of others in the group. Therefore, you handle creative decision-making very well. In high-control situations, you become bored; in low-control situations, you become overly concerned with getting group support, often at the expense of the job at hand. You don't like high stress situations.

If you are a **low LPC leader** (if you scored 57 or less), you are a task-motivated, no-nonsense leader. You are more concerned with the job to be done for the association than with getting the association's support. You are eager and often impatient to get on with the work. In high-control situations, you can relax because the job is under control; you can take time to develop good relations with others in the group. As long as the work gets done, you are happy. You are also effective in low-control situations. Under pressure, you organize and direct the group to finish the task. You control the group tightly with strict discipline. You are not as successful in moderate-control situations. There is often group conflict that you cannot control. You are insensitive to others' feelings, and the group resents that. You work best with guidelines and specific directions.

If you are a **moderate LPC leader** (if you scored between 58 and 63), your style is not clear. You need to determine which style fits best with your approaches.

A **high-control situation** is one in which the leader has a predictable environment, the support of the group, a well-defined and highly structured task, and power; he or she must be diplomatic. There is no conflict.

A **moderate-control situation** is one in which the task may be ambiguous. The leader is concerned about the group's feelings, is possibly in a weak position of power, and must be diplomatic. The leader works around conflict.

A **low-control situation** is challenging and difficult, with an unstructured task, a non-supportive group, and a weak position of power for the leader. The leader takes control of any conflict that may exist.

Figure 1–2

LEADERSHIP STYLE TEST

(Douglas 1992)

The following 20 statements relate to your ideal image of leadership. As you respond to them, imagine yourself to be a leader and then answer the questions in a way that would reflect your particular style of leadership. It makes no difference what kind of leadership experience, if any, you have had or are currently involved in. The purpose is to establish your ideal preference for relating with subordinates.

The format includes a five-point scale, ranging from **Strongly Agree** to **Strongly Disagree** for each statement. Select one point on each scale and mark it as you read the 20 statements relating to leadership. You may omit answers to questions that are confusing or that you feel you cannot answer.

	STRONGLY AGREE	AGREE	MIXED FEELINGS	DISAGREE	STRONGLY DISAGREE
1. When I tell a subordinate to do something, I expect them to do it with no questions asked. After all, I am responsible for what they do.	1	2	3	4	5
2. Tight control by a leader usually does more harm than good. People will generally do the best job when they are allowed to exercise self-control.	5	4	3	2	1
3. Although discipline is important in an organization, the effective leader should mediate the use of disciplinary procedures with his/her knowledge of the people and the situation.	1	2	3	4	5
4. A leader must make every effort to subdivide the tasks of the people to the greatest possible extent.	1	2	3	4	5
5. Shared leadership or truly democratic process in a group can work only when a recognized leader assists the process.	1	2	3	4	5

7

6. As a leader, I am ultimately responsible for all of the actions of my group. If our activities result in benefits for the organization, I should be rewarded accordingly.	1	2	3	4	5
7. To do a good job, most persons require only minimum direction from their leader .	5	4	3	2	1
8. Subordinates usually require the control of a strict leader.	1	2	3	4	5
9. Leadership can be shared among participants of a group, so that at any one time the group could have two or more leaders.	5	4	3	2	1
10. Leadership should generally come from the top, but there are some logical exceptions to this rule.	5	4	3	2	1
11. The disciplinary function of the leader is simply to seek democratic opinions on problems as they arise.	5	4	3	2	1
12. The engineering problems, the management time, and the worker frustration caused by the division of labor are hardly ever worth the savings. In most cases, workers are most effective at determining their own job content.	5	4	3	2	1
13. A group's leader should be the member whom the other members elect to coordinate their activities and represent them to the rest of the organization.	5	4	3	2	1

14. A leader needs to exercise some control over the people.	1	2	3	4	5
15. There must be one and only one recognized leader in a group.	1	2	3	4	5
16. A good leader must establish and strictly enforce an impersonal system of discipline.	1	2	3	4	5
17. Discipline codes should be flexible and should allow the leader to make individual decisions in each particular situation.	5	4	3	2	1
18. Basically, people are responsible for themselves and no one else. Thus, a leader cannot be blamed or take credit for the work of subordinates.	5	4	3	2	1
19. The job of the leader is to relate a task to subordinates, ask them for ways in which it can best be accomplished, and help them reach a consensus on a plan of attack.	5	4	3	2	1
20. If people are in a position of leadership, it is assumed that they are generally superior to their workers.	1	2	3	4	5

SCORING

You may score your own leadership style by averaging the numbers that correspond to your answer for each individual item. For example, if you answered "Strongly Agree" to the first item, your score for that item would be "1". To obtain your overall leadership style, add all of the numerical values that are associated with the 20 leadership items and divide by 20. The resulting average is your leadership style.

INTERPRETATIONS

SCORE	DESCRIPTION	LEADERSHIP STYLE
1.9 or lower	Very Autocratic	Boss decides and announces decisions, rules, orientation
2.0–2.4	Moderately Autocratic	Boss announces decisions but asks for questions, makes exceptions to rules
2.5–3.4	Mixed	Boss suggests ideas and consults groups; many exceptions to regulations
3.5–4.0	Moderately Participative	Group decides on basis of boss' suggestions; rules are few; group proceeds as they see fit
4.1 or higher	Very Democratic	Group is in charge of decisions; boss is coordinator; group makes any rules

THEORIES OF LEADERSHIP

- ◆ Great Man Theory
- ◆ Trait Theory
- ◆ Situational Theory
- ◆ Modern Theories

TASKS OF LEADERSHIP

(Gardner 1989)

- ◆ Envisioning Goals — *pointing others in the right direction, dealing c̄ tensions*
- ◆ Affirming Values *vision beliefs, values purpose revitalize*
- ◆ Motivating *channeling motives challenge*

- ◆ Managing *plan, set priorities make decisions*
- ◆ Achieving a Workable Unity *trust cohesion tolerance manage conflict loyalty*
- ◆ Explaining *helping others understand the vision*
- ◆ Serving as a Symbol *of hope voice of anger, risk taking source collective identity*
- ◆ Representing the Group *advocating*

- ◆ Renewing *blending continuity & change*

DEVELOPING AND RENEWING OTHERS

- Personal Attention
- Role Modeling
- Precepting
- Mentoring

NOTES

THE NEW WORLD AND NEW LEADERSHIP...

CHANGING OUR THINKING ABOUT LEADERSHIP

2

Nurses must set a standard of excellence for themselves and accept responsibility for influencing change in healthcare. To accomplish these goals, nurses must gain self-confidence. This can be achieved by becoming competent in creating new strategies to provide healthcare, using scarce resources wisely, participating in developing healthcare policy, and partnering with others. Nurses must begin to think differently about the broader delivery of care and must not focus merely on the provision of direct patient care. Nurses must be involved in writing grants, networking with community agencies, sharing expertise and resources, preparing educational materials, and assisting in establishing health policy. In other words, they must function as leaders.

Leadership is the key to changing from a task orientation to a professional orientation and to a patient outcome focus. It also is the key to equal collaboration of nursing with other healthcare disciplines. Nurses can no longer be handmaidens to others, blindly accepting orders and carrying them out. Those of us in the nursing field must define what nurses do and what we want nurses to do; we must then work as a unified body to achieve our goals.

The current "whitewater" chaos of healthcare needs to be viewed as challenging and invigorating, not as overwhelming and depressing. Such chaos actually gives nursing an opportunity to embrace "a piece of the healthcare pie" — a piece that is our own, in which nurses truly nurse patients and do not merely follow physicians' orders. Our profession has already grabbed a piece of this pie by defining advanced nursing practice, in which nurses diagnose, prescribe, evaluate, and consult with physicians in delivering primary, secondary, and tertiary care.

Perhaps Wheatley (1992, 20) said it best when she stated that "growth is found in disequilibrium, not in balance". According to the new science, living systems organize themselves by seeking order, but this order is not linear and predictive. Quantum theory suggests that an interface among all members of a group is critical. People need to be given the opportunity to grow in all kinds of ways — ways that are unknown to anyone until they happen. This new way of thinking about leadership in a global and limitless fashion acknowledges that each individual has a contribution to make. Porter-O'Grady (1997) reminds us that we have to use our imaginations and be more accepting of the idea that our work involves more than assessing, planning, implementing, and evaluating. We need to adapt the "New Science of Leadership" (Wheatley 1992), with its focus on empowering followers and alleviating bureaucratic structures, so that we can develop new ideas and new ways of thinking.

OBJECTIVES

♦ Define the new leadership that nurses must adopt in order to participate successfully in and shape the healthcare system of today and tomorrow.

♦ Examine how chaos creates new opportunities for nurses to function as leaders in the healthcare delivery system.

♦ Describe how each of the following is congruent with the new leadership: quantum theory, developmental theory, cognitive theory, and perspective transformation theory.

♦ Identify how the new leadership influences the nursing profession as well as individual nurses throughout their careers.

♦ Describe strategies to assist nurses' development as new leaders.

KEY WORDS

Chaos Theory

New Leadership/ New Science of Leadership

Quantum Theory

Scientific Age/ Industrial Age/Newtonian Age

ACTIVITIES

1. Have the students identify individuals who, in their opinion, exhibit the kind of leadership described in the text. Encourage students to include individuals who have a local, national, and international impact. Ask students to use these individuals as "role model leaders" and to propose how the units or agencies where they practice could embody this new way of thinking about leadership: What would the nurse manager need to do differently to be more like the "role model leaders" identified? What would staff need to do in order to begin to function like these "role model" leaders?

2. Students will need to be articulate and assertive in expressing their views on this new way of leading. Some nurses will need assertiveness training to change from handmaiden to autonomous provider. Review assertive, non-assertive, and aggressive behaviors. Have students divide into groups of four. Randomly assign each student in each group to model the nurse manager or a nurse demonstrating assertive, non-assertive, or aggressive behavior. After 5 to 10 minutes of role playing, ask each group to share with the entire class their experiences (a) as the individual acting in an assertive, non-assertive, or aggressive manner, and (b) as the "recipient" of different types of behavior. Compare the experiences of each group and relate the findings to methods of functioning as a leader.

3. Using a scenario similar to that provided in Figure 2–1, have groups of students (four or –five to a group) develop three ways (using assertive, nonassertive, and aggressive behavior) in which the scenario could evolve. After 10 minutes of group work, ask each group to report the "results" of each type of encounter. If desired, students could take a course on intensive assertiveness training through the university or local adult education program.

4. There is no question that staff nurses in hospital and home care settings face tremendous challenges. Have the students break into small groups, assign each group one scenario from Figure 2–2, and propose ways in which using the "New Science of Leadership" could facilitate some successful solutions to these situations. After allowing students to work for 15 minutes, have the groups return to the larger class. Each group's delegated recorder should then share the group's findings with the class and discuss the classes' suggestions.

REFERENCES

Porter-O'Grady, T. 1997. Quantum mechanics and the future of healthcare leadership. *Journal of Nursing Administration* 27:15–20.

Wheatley, M. 1992. *Leadership and the new science: Learning about organization from an orderly universe.* San Francisco: Berrett-Koehler Publishers.

Figure 2–1

SCENARIO FOR APPLICATION OF ASSERTIVE, NON-ASSERTIVE, AND AGGRESSIVE BEHAVIOR

Sue Brown, RN, a critical care staff nurse with 4 years of experience, just had a problem with one of the new resident physicians. The resident was inserting a pulmonary catheter, and Sue notified him that the patient was in ventricular fibrillation. Sue also told him that according to the hemodynamic waveform, the catheter had cleared the right ventricle and was now in the pulmonary artery. The physician answered, "Don't worry about a little ventricular fibrillation... it's expected after right ventricular irritation. You know, you should know this. Haven't you ever assisted anyone with a pulmonary catheter insertion?" Sue repeated that the patient was in ventricular fibrillation, and the physician laughed and said, "Don't you think you are getting carried away?" Sue repeated herself again and defibrillated the patient, who responded. The physician said nothing, cleared the bed after two commands, and simply walked away. The patient was stable. Sue notified the patient's attending physician, the medical director of the intensive care unit, and her nurse manager.

Hypothesize ways in which Sue can be *assertive*, *nonassertive*, and *aggressive* in managing this conflict.

Figure 2–2

TYPICAL STAFF NURSE ASSIGNMENT SCENARIOS:

HOME CARE AND HOSPITAL

1. Mr. Coone is a patient who is visited at his home regularly. His blood glucose level is 450–500 mg/dL in the late afternoon/evening and plummets to 40–50 mg/dL by early morning. The primary physician orders regular humulin insulin, using a different scale each time. The nurse does not have confidence in asking why Mr. Coone isn't on ultralente insulin every morning or why a consistent sliding scale couldn't be used. In fact, the nurse does not even recognize that both of these questions are totally relevant and that both should be explored so that adequate care can be given to this patient.

2. Ms. Meisner, a 32-year-old, is spitting up about 10 mL of bright red blood approximately every 15 minutes. Her diagnosis is cystic fibrosis. She has an indwelling venous access device for administration of her antibiotics and steroids. The pulmonologist initially explains that the hemoptysis is secondary to scar tissue from the disease process; he says it is expected in patients with long-standing cystic fibrosis. Ms. Meisner's vital signs are stable and do not reflect hypovolemia, so her condition is not considered life threatening at this time. Orders include vital signs every half hour, oxygen as needed with increased nebulizer treatments, CBC stat, and bed rest. When Ms. Meisner's blood pressure decreases, the nurse notifies the house officer on call, who orders an increased rate of intravenous fluid and refuses to come up and see the patient. The house officer also asks that she not be called again about this patient and tells the nurse, "I think she is sucking blood out of her Port-A-Cath and then spitting it up for attention."

3. It is 8:00 a.m. and your patient, Mrs. Tye, is scheduled for a CAT scan at 2:00 p.m. Mrs. Tye has encephalopathy secondary to diabetic coma post-delivery. Her total parenteral nutrition (TPN) was stopped at midnight, as ordered, in preparation for the study. Her blood glucose level is now 42 mg/dL. She has orders for 15 units of NPH insulin daily. Her doctor is not responding to the page, so the nurse is faced with several questions: Should he give dextrose? Restart the TPN? Hold the NPH insulin order? Records indicate that Mrs. Tye has not been this hypoglycemic previously.

4. Mrs. Soot, 78-years-old, asks why her visitors and the staff have to put on gowns before entering her room. She wonders how she has acquired vancomycin-resistant enterococci (VRE) in her stool when she was admitted for an exacerbation of her congestive heart failure. She also inquires why the patient care coordinator asked her if she was familiar with a different long-term care facility than the one from which she came. She says, "I have been at Green Valley for about 2 years now, and I have several friends there. I know all of the staff there so, of course, I want to go back there. They are holding my bed and room for me." The nurse notices that Mrs. Soot is tachycardic and also dyspneic and is getting really "worked up" about this conversation. The nurse, therefore, does not tell Mrs. Soot that she will probably have to transfer to a different facility because Green Valley does not accept VRE patients.

5. Mr. Jones's blood pressure is 90/58 mm Hg, well below his normal reading, and over the past 4 hours it has decreased from 148/84 mm Hg. He is not urinating much (60 mL during the past 4 hours), and he is not drinking. His lungs are clear, but the nurse is not absolutely sure whether the lung sounds are diminished posteriorly. Mr. Jones is only 28 years old and has recently received a diagnosis of

Crohn's disease. The home care nurse feels that he should be hospitalized, but she is unable to reach his primary provider.

6. Mr. Dootie, a 33-year–old patient with AIDS, has a CD4 count of 33 cells/mm^3 and an RNA viral load less than 900,000 copies/mL. He has experienced at least 20 opportunistic infections over the past 6 months. He says, "I am more afraid of prolonging my dying than of death itself." He is getting ready to leave the hospital against medical advice.

SUPPORTING PERSPECTIVES FOR
THE NEW SCIENCE OF LEADERSHIP

- Cognitive/Intellectual Development

- Developmental Theory

- Perspective Transformation

NOTES

22

FOLLOWERSHIP AND EMPOWERMENT

3

INTRODUCTION

Followership is a skill that can be learned, just as leadership can be learned. Followers are expected to support leaders by asking questions, giving thoughtful feedback, working to achieve group goals, and providing encouragement when the leader takes a risk on behalf of the group.

Sadly, however, followers are often thought of as passive, unthinking individuals who merely go along with whatever the leader suggests. Because of this kind of perspective, it is not surprising that many individuals are not particularly excited about being thought of as followers. The role of follower, however, is essential to the success of any endeavor. Without followers, leaders are powerless.

It is important to realize that effective followers have many of the same characteristics as effective leaders, including strength; accountability; independence; critical thinking; an ability and willingness to think for oneself; give honest feedback, be innovative, be creative, be cooperative, go "above and beyond;" collaborate; a tendency to be a self-starter; and a sense of being energized by one's work. In other words, there is little to apologize for when one is an effective follower.

However, like most other individuals, nurses are not socialized to think of themselves as effective followers who have some degree of power in situations. But they *are* quite powerful. For example, a leader can express a vision, but that vision will remain a dream and will never become reality without the support and investment of followers. In addition, leaders may carefully outline phases of moving from one type of practice to another, but without the work of followers, such a change will never occur.

Rather than thinking of themselves as passive "sheep" who are expected merely to go along with whatever plans others outline—whether it is a plan of care outlined by a physician, a new staffing plan outlined by the nurse manager, or a plan for working with unlicensed assistants outlined by the hospital administration--- nurses need to think of themselves as individuals who have the right and responsibility to question and challenge those plans. Taking on the role of effective follower, however, is not easy.

Nurses who wish to be effective followers need to be aware of their own strengths and abilities; have a degree of self confidence; and know how to question, when to question, and who to question. They need to feel empowered, as if they have something significant to offer. They also need to accept that being an effective follower is just as critical to creating a preferred future for nursing as being an effective leader. Leaders are leaders only if they have followers. Followers need to use their power wisely.

OBJECTIVES

♦ Analyze the concept of followership.

♦ Examine elements of the follower role that are appealing and those that are not.

♦ Examine the similarities between leaders and followers.

♦ Articulate the interdependence between leaders and followers.

♦ Formulate strategies to develop oneself as an effective follower.

KEY WORDS

Advocate	Enlightened Followers	Power
Apathy	Followership	Stewardship
Collaboration	Leadership	"Yes" People
Credibility	Networking	
Empowerment	Partnership	

ACTIVITIES

1. Divide students into groups of four and direct them to role-play a contemporary work situation (Figure 3–1). Each person in the group should depict one of the four types of followers described by Kelley (1992): sheep, exemplary follower, alienated follower, and "yes" person. The instructor can act as the nurse manager. Be sure to have the class identify the unattractive as well as the attractive characteristics of each type of follower. Have another group of four students role-play the same work situation using Pittman, Rosenbach, and Potter's (1998) followership styles: partner, contributor, politician, and subordinate; the instructor should again play the role of nurse manager. Examine how these roles are similar to or different from Kelly's, discuss how effective/exemplary followers or partners can be developed and encouraged, and explore the extent to which each student fulfills the role of effective/exemplary follower or partner in a group.

2. Assign each student to a 4 to 6–hour apprenticeship, such as the following: working with affiliating agency personnel in developing a grant proposal, planning a health fair with the local community health agency, participating in preparing for a Joint Commission on Accreditation of Healthcare Organizations visit, "shadowing" a nurse member of the State Board of Nurse Examiners, observing the executive officer of the State Nurses Association or National League for Nursing for a day, or participating in any other activity the student feels would be an interesting opportunity to practice what a leader does. In a written assignment, students should analyze the person's role as a nurse leader and follower and explain how the student, as a follower, incorporated at least 10 of the listed strategies of effective following (Figure 3–2).

3. Have the class write an article for the alumni, Student Nurses Association, or Sigma Theta Tau chapter newsletter. A large class can be broken into 3 groups, with each group writing an article for a different publication. The article should examine the similarities between leaders and

followers and the interdependence that exists between them and should be directed toward the audience for each publication.

4. Using a clinical situation that involves staff nurses, have the students apply Chaleff's (1995) perception of leaders and followers both orbiting around a purpose (Text Figure 3–1) rather than the conventional idea of followers orbiting around the leader. Be sure to emphasize the significance of the power held by staff nurses who are effective followers, even though they do not officially have authority.

5. Propose two specific strategies one could use to increase one's political astuteness (and, thereby, one's power base) in the institution where one is working or will work. Students can use strategies from Figure 3-2. Discuss the significance of empowering oneself in order to have the self-confidence to feel competent.

6. Have the students complete the Followership Style Test (Text Display 3–1) before class and then share their followership styles in small groups. Explain the relations among followership styles (autocratic, mixed, and democratic) and styles of leadership (laissez-faire, democratic, and autocratic). Have the students propose hypothetical situations that would be appropriate for each of the noted styles of leadership and followership.

7. Have students use Figure 3–3, "How to Test Your Delegation Habits" (Krein 1982), to determine how well they are delegating. In small groups, discuss options (including the strategies of becoming a more effective follower) that could increase ability to delegate. Have students pair up (one with high delegation skills and one with lower delegation skills) to role-play delegating. Students with low delegation skills could re-take "How to Test Your Delegation Habits" after practicing.

REFERENCES

Chaleff, I. 1995. *The courageous follower: Standing up to and for our leaders*. San Francisco: Berrett-Koehler Publishers.

Kelley, R. 1992. *The power of followership: How to create leaders people want to follow and followers who lead themselves*. New York: Doubleday Currency.

Krein, T. 1982. How to improve delegation habits. *Management Review* 71:58–61.

Pittman, T., W. Rosenbach, and E. Potter. 1998. Followers as partners: Taking the initiative for action. In *Contemporary issues in leadership*. 4th ed., 107–120. Edited by W. Rosenbach and R. Taylor. Boulder, CO: Westview Press.

Figure 3–1

CONTEMPORARY WORK SITUATION

A nurse manager with an impressive track record, who is new to the institution but has 3 years of experience as a nurse manager of a comparable unit, hires seven new graduates to fill vacancies. The general feeling is that the previous nurse manager had no pride in the unit and was just "putting in her time before retirement;" therefore, several of the more recently hired RNs (i.e., those who had spent less than 2 years on the unit) had transferred to other units. The vice president for nursing worked with the remaining nurses to select this new nurse manager, and as a result, most of the staff is very supportive of working as a team with the manager on improving morale and productivity. Given this information, determine how the leader and followers on this unit can succeed in orienting and retaining the new graduates.

Figure 3–2

STRATEGIES TO USE

TO BECOME AN EFFECTIVE FOLLOWER

- Be involved in one's practice setting

- Continue one's education

- Take initiative

- Be committed to something other than one's own career development

- Know one's organization

- Know one's own values and hold on to them

- Set a standard that demonstrates high values

- Be involved in professional organizations

- Seek out mentors or be a mentor

- Feel free to criticize, but do not just complain and walk away

- Be proactive; advocate and be a catalyst for change

- Remain fully accountable for one's actions

- Be reflective

- Develop one's professional networks

- Share information rather than horde it

- Help colleagues grow and do their job well

- Have a sense of humor and laugh at one's own mistakes

Figure 3–3

HOW TO TEST YOUR DELEGATION HABITS

(Krein 1992)

Directions: Choose Strongly Agree (5), Agree (4), Do Not Have an Opinion (3), Disagree (2), or Strongly Disagree (1) for each of the following statements. Add up all of the scores and compare them to the scoring guidelines noted below.

_____ 1. I'd delegate more, but the jobs I delegate never seem to get done the way I want them to be done.

_____ 2. I don't feel I have the time to delegate properly.

_____ 3. I carefully check on subordinates' work without letting them know I'm doing it, so I can correct their mistakes if necessary before they cause too many problems.

_____ 4. I delegate the whole job, giving the opportunity for the subordinate to complete it without any of my involvement. Then I review the end result.

_____ 5. When I have given clear instructions and the job isn't done right, I get upset.

_____ 6. I feel the staff lacks the commitment that I have. Any job I delegate won't get done as well as I'd do it.

_____ 7. I'd delegate more, but I feel that I can do the task better than the person I might delegate it to.

_____ 8. I'd delegate more, but if the individual I delegate the task to does an incompetent job, I'll be severely criticized.

_____ 9. If I were to delegate the task, my job wouldn't be nearly as much fun.

_____ 10. When I delegate a job, I often find that the outcome is such that I end up doing the job over again myself.

_____ 11. I have not really found that delegation saves any time.

_____ 12. I delegate a task clearly and concisely, explaining exactly how it should be accomplished.

_____ 13. I can't delegate as much as I'd like to because my subordinates lack the necessary experience.

_____ 14. I feel that when I delegate, I lose control.

_____ 15. I would delegate more, but I'm pretty much a perfectionist.

_____ 16. I work longer hours than I should.

_____ 17. I can give subordinates the routine tasks, but I feel I must keep non-routine tasks myself.

_____ 18. My own boss expects me to keep very close to all details of the work.

Scoring Guidelines

A score between *72 and 90* means you are not delegating correctly at all.

A score between *54 and 71* means your delegating needs substantial improvement .A score between *36 and 53* means you could improve but are definitely delegating.

A score between *0 and 35* means you are delegating very well.

TYPES OF FOLLOWERS

(Kelley, 1992)

- ◆ Effective or Exemplary Followers

- ◆ Alienated Followers

- ◆ "Yes" People

- ◆ Sheep

DIMENSIONS OF FOLLOWERSHIP STYLES

(Pittman, Rosenbach, and Potter 1998)

- ◆ Partner

- ◆ Contributor

- ◆ Politician

- ◆ Subordinate

NOTES

LEADERSHIP AS AN INTEGRAL COMPONENT OF A PROFESSIONAL ROLE

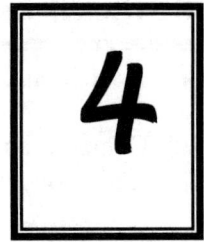

4

INTRODUCTION

Collaboration is imperative in order to ensure quality patient care that does not involve duplication or fragmentation and offers a more holistic perspective and a shared responsibility for the well-being of the patient. Before nurses can collaborate effectively, however, it is important for us to know our professional role and how that role fits in as an integral part of a team structure. Barriers of the past must be broke down so nurses can have the opportunity to provide autonomous and accountable patient care.

Nurses are the biggest group of healthcare providers. It is paramount that nurses be prepared for our ever-expanding role so that our numbers can be used to our advantage. Gone are the days when competent bedside patient care was the ultimate goal of novice nurses. Today's nurses must be prepared to practice competently within a broad frame of reference and must have a much more telescopic, rather than microscopic, perspective. For example, nurses not only need to identify patients with health problems but should also be able to negotiate the financial support necessary to provide for these populations, prepare evidence-based nursing practice protocols to implement and evaluate appropriate care, develop health teaching programs for individuals anywhere along the wellness-illness continuum, establish and implement quality improvement standards, lobby for safe practice, and spearhead various other strategic moves to improve patient care. No longer can activities such as these be thought of as the purview of other healthcare professionals.

Transformational leadership is defined by Burns (1978) as a process by which leaders and followers rise together, cohesively, to high levels of motivation. It is this underlying motivation that empowers a group or an organization to succeed. Transactional leadership, which involves an exchange in which both the leader and follower receive "something" as they accomplish the task, is not enough. Leadership in today's and tomorrow's world must be transformational.

Communication ability is an aspect of leadership that can help create a more transformational leader. It is paramount that all communications be clear and understandable, accomplish the purpose for having the communication, and get to the right people. As a leader, one must be able to communicate well enough to influence or motivate others to set and achieve group goals. It is interesting to note that one-half of any speaker's message is a result of his or her facial and body language/. Therefore, the need to maintain professional dress, demeanor, and semantics is critical. It is often said that a person feels as good as he or she looks. If this is true, and it certainly seems to be, nurses need to be conscious of consistently depicting a professional image.

OBJECTIVES

♦ Identify characteristics of transformational and transactional leaders.

♦ Compare and contrast the leader/follower relationship in a transformational environment and the leader/follower relationship in a transactional environment.

♦ Explain how transformational leadership generates growth in an individual, organization, or group.

♦ Describe how Maslow's hierarchy of needs relates to leadership development.

♦ Explain how leadership is an integral component of each professional nurse's role.

KEY WORDS

Behavioral Objectives	Empowerment	Organizational Culture
Collaboration	Group Process	Participative Management
Conflict Management	Hardiness	Transactional Leadership
Decentralization	Leadership	Transformational Leadership
Effective Presentation	Maslow's Hierarchy	Vision

ACTIVITIES

1. Have students analyze the scenarios on conflict management in Figure 4-1. Review the type of conflict, the ways in which to resolve the conflict, and the mediation used to resolve the conflict (confrontation, bargaining, smoothing, avoidance, and forcing). Use Figure 4-2, "Management of Conflict," to review strategies used in dealing with conflict.

2. To demonstrate how nursing interventions have improved patient outcomes, professional nurses must be able to plan and evaluate care. .In addition, nurses who teach patients should include measurable criteria that participants must achieve. Have the students develop behavioral objectives for teaching individual patients in the acute care setting and groups in a community setting. Behavioral objectives should list the desired behavior, the evaluation method used to measure whether the behavior has been accomplished, and the target time/date for completion of the behavior. Be sure to differentiate learner activities from participant behaviors. For example, a student may market a program by putting up posters advertising the day and time of the session (a learner activity) but should mainly focus on the degree to which participants in the program actually learned (participant behavior).

3. Some institutions that have experienced downsizing are now applying transformational leadership. Using the Shadyside Hospital Model (see Text Chapter 4 and Figure 4-3), have the students work in small groups to identify how their unit or agency may need to be changed in terms of staff morale, job satisfaction, and patient outcomes if the staff were to exhibit hardiness, empowerment, and vision and if the organization were to undergo total decentralization, develop

a new organizational culture, and implement participative management. Students should propose at least five advantages of adapting transformational leadership that would benefit their unit or agency.

4. Give the students tasks to solve, such as determining how to market a new outpatient intravenous therapy program or developing a policy or protocol for a medication algorithm to be used in the ventilated anxious versus agitated patient. The focus of this assignment is to accomplish the task with maximum involvement of all group members. Have the students share the strategies that have helped their group to work cohesively and to accomplish their tasks. Assist them in understanding that leaders must help groups proceed through forming, storming, norming, and performing stages before they can accomplish their task.

REFERENCES

Burns, J. 1978. *Leadership*. New York: Harper & Row.

Covey, S. 1989. *Seven habits of highly effective people*. New York: Fireside.

Kuntzleman, C. 1992. *Maximizing your energy and personal productivity*. Chaska, MN: Nordic Press.

Figure 4–1

CONFLICT MANAGEMENT SCENARIOS

Scenario 1: Your nurse manager often validates the narcotic count with the pharmacy technician when the PYXIS machine is filled. You have noted on three separate occasions that the narcotic total does not match what is in the machine. All three occasions have occurred very soon after the nurse manager and the pharmacy technician filled the PYXIS. Your actions include ....

Scenario 2: As a nurse manager, you are faced with scheduling the staff for the Thanksgiving, Christmas, and New Year's Day holidays. The unit has no policy on this scheduling, which has always been a nightmare that everyone has somehow lived through. There are 35 RNs and 10 unlicensed assistive personnel (UAP). You expect a full census, and closing beds is not an option. How would you proceed?

Scenario 3: You have just been promoted to nurse manager of the ICU. You have worked in the unit for 6 years and enjoy a good relationship with all of the staff. In fact, three of the 17 RNs are your best friends. One of your friends is pregnant and has asked for special assignments during her pregnancy. You realize that such "favoring" has not been done in the past for pregnant nurses. You plan to be proactive about this potential problem. What is your plan?

Scenario 4: As per **Scenario 3** above, one of your other friends has asked to go to a 3-day conference and has applied for tuition reimbursement. Yesterday, another nurse applied to go to this same conference. According to unit policy, only one nurse can be sent to a particular conference. How will you resolve this dilemma?

Scenario 5: You have just finished assisting with a pulmonary artery catheter insertion on your patient. The physician retorts, "This was a tough insertion, and I cannot believe you did not have the defibrillator charged and at the bedside in case we needed it. You are just plain lucky this time. I suppose stupid people do tend to be lucky!" This physician is new to the intensive care unit and was not aware that she should have requested the defibrillator if she felt it was necessary. How will you respond to her?

Figure 4–2

MANAGEMENT OF CONFLICT

- Clarify communications... Be open, honest

- Avoid taking sides… Try to reserve judgment until the issue is clear

- Avoid highly emotional and unfair confrontations

- Work toward congruence between role and status

- Work toward congruence among power, authority, and competence

- Engage in reconciliation

- Employ problem-solving skills

- Engage in compromise

- Work toward mutual alliances... common pacts

- Go on strike… Engage in arbitration

- Develop needed skills

- Identify the source of the conflict

- Participate in integrative decision-making

Figure 4–3

THE TRANSFORMATIONAL MODEL:

STAFF AND ORGANIZATION CONCEPTS

STAFF CONCEPTS

    Hardiness

    Empowerment

    Vision

ORGANIZATION CONCEPTS

    Participative Decentralization

    Management

    Organizational Culture

Operating System

PRACTICES THAT TRANSFORM FOLLOWERS

(Kuntzelman, 1992)

- ♦ Challenge the status quo

- ♦ Inspire a shared vision

- ♦ Enable others to act, rather than to react

- ♦ Be a role model

- ♦ Encourage the heart

SEVEN HABITS OF
HIGHLY EFFECTIVE PEOPLE

(Covey, 1989)

- Be proactive

- Begin with the end (goal) in mind

- Put first things first

- Think win/win

- Seek first to understand... then to be understood

- Synergize

- Sharpen the saw (be proactive about the future)

VISION AND CREATIVITY 5

It is important that students realize that each of us needs a vision, or inner core of values, that guides us in making decisions about and throughout life. These values or commitments must be sacred; in other words, they must not change no matter what challenges one faces in life, even challenges that are made to one's values themselves.

One individual, for example, may have a strong sense of family pride and may choose to maintain that bond by frequently telephoning geographically distant family members, arranging periodic visits, maintaining traditional "get-togethers" or other family "rituals," and helping family members whenever necessary. Maintaining family closeness is paramount to this individual, and she will "schedule" family-related activities into her life. Therefore, although she may not be geographically close to her family, she makes it a point to follow through with this commitment. Such a value may influence this individual's work situation because she may appreciate the family responsibilities of others and may make allowances for absences from work, inability to complete a project in a very short period of time, or unwillingness to travel far from home on business. Valuing the maintenance of family ties will have an impact on the individual's entire life, including where her family resides, how her work is perceived, how her leisure time is spent, and the general way that her life is lived. It will also affect how she participates in the work organization and how seriously she commits to the organization's philosophy, mission, and overall strategic plan.

Values such as these translate into visions. Vision encompasses one's core values, which are more immediate, as well as one's future-oriented dreams. Each of us needs to hold onto our core values while we learn to get away from routine, specific, step-by-step, potentially restricting frames of reference and instead imagine ways in which the group, profession, or organization with which we are involved can grow and evolve. By seeing our core values as the basis for much-sought-after dreams, we may better understand what a vision really is and how it can help us accomplish our goals.

Greenleaf (cited in Spears 1998) advanced the idea that visions crystallize when people, in ordinary conversation, say things to each other that are related to dreams or feelings they share . He points out that this type of conversation occurs when people are committed and, often, when they are in high-performing, forward-looking organizations. Basically, Greenleaf highlights the importance of people working together to create and achieve mutual goals rather than a single individual competing for self-recognition and reward.

It also is important for each of us to use our creativity if we are to be successful "dreamers" or "vision-creators" and, therefore, successful and actualized leaders. In the creative, visioning process, everyone's perspective has merit and there is no one "right" idea. Nurses and nursing students should use their own ideas when providing nursing care, be creative, and work toward realizing their vision of excellence in practice, not merely do what others have done or prescribed. Who better to develop such creative ideas than nursing's future leaders, our students?

OBJECTIVES

- Define the concept of a vision as it relates to leadership.

- Describe how a nurse leader or follower can facilitate the identification, articulation, and communication of a personal vision.

- Identify strategies that would be effective in making one's personal vision a reality.

- Formulate a personal vision for the profession or one's particular area of practice.

- Identify characteristics of nursing and non-nursing leaders who are viewed as visionary.

- Describe characteristics of a creative person, process, and environment.

- Project potential outcomes of using creativity as a nurse leader or follower.

- Identify how the new science of leadership fosters an individual's creativity to improve leadership and followership.

- Examine how the incorporation of vision and creativity into the profession can help vitalize/energize a nurse.

KEY WORDS

Change	Entrepreneur	Strategic Plan
Communication	Mission	Systems Thinker
Creativity	Persuasion	Vision
Critical Path	Philosophy	Visionary
Empowerment	Power	

ACTIVITIES

1. Use Conger's "Typology of Visions" (Text Figure 5-1) to categorize a healthcare agency's vision as externally or internally oriented and narrow or broad in perspective. Review a copy of the agency's annual report and discuss how the agency's mission, philosophy, and strategic plan are affected by its vision.

2. Have the students divide into groups of eight and direct them to imagine how they, as nurses, could develop a vision for their unit or department. Use Kouzes and Posner's (1993) "Eight-Point Framework" (Figure 5-1) as a guide. Explain to the students that they have the knowledge and expertise to identify what is really important and what should be kept "sacred;" explain how this

knowledge shapes an agency's growth and future. The groups should tell the class their conclusions and their recommendations on ways to communicate their vision to the unit or department and to other areas of the agency.

3. Identify how the "road blocking" experienced by the APRNs at the inner city clinic (Text Chapter 5) actually expanded the nurses' scope of practice and the mission of the clinic beyond the originally developed vision.

4. Ask the students to share their ideas of how individuals like Bill Gates and Mother Theresa gained the power to lead through their extraordinary visions. Discuss the types of power that people have, such as referent, legitimate, expert, coercive and reward, and have students share their sources of power. Then ask them to discuss how these sources of power can help them do extraordinary things in achieving their visions. Be sure to discuss how limiting oneself is more detrimental to realizing one's visions than life's challenges and barriers, and discuss how most people do not use 90% of their inherent potential. Use the example of the mountain climber (Wood 1995), who said that the real fight was not with the mountain but with her mind, and that once she decided to commit to finishing the climb, she realized that she was the one who had been creating the barriers.

5. Using the motivation theories of McGregor, Herzberg, and Maslow, have all students explain how vision can be enhanced in themselves and in their peers. Introduce the term *hardiness*, which is often associated with the Transformational Leadership Theory, and discuss how one's inner core of values, or vision, influences one's desire to follow through, work hard, and generally be accountable for one's actions.

6. Hold class outside or in another setting, or create a different classroom environment by bringing in posters, paintings, displays, or music. After using brainstorming or mindmapping to get students to share their ideas about various issues related to practice, ask them to develop a different type of patient contract; write an ideal job description for a nurse; or design a delivery system that would allow truly professional nursing practice and, at the same time, maximize patient outcomes.

7. Review the excerpt from Wheatley and Kellnor-Rogers' book, *A Simpler Way* (1996), about how life creates itself. Divide the class into seven groups, and assign each group one of the beliefs about life. After 20 minutes, ask each group to apply "their" belief to a realistic practice problem and to develop a workable solution and a plan to evaluate the effectiveness of their proposed solution. Then ask students to explain how they can create a work environment that is energizing, challenging, rewarding, and growth-producing.

8. Using the How Creative Are You checklist (Text Display 5.3), ask the students to determine their level of creativity. Hypothesize how individuals can enhance their ability to be creative.

9. Ask students to bring to class a written description of their own visions of their practice in 5 to 10 years, ways in which their units or agencies can function more effectively, and the future of the nursing profession. Discuss with the entire class the things that would need to be done to realize each student's vision.

REFERENCES

Kouzes, J., and B. Posner. 1993. *Credibility.* San Francisco: Jossey-Bass.

Spears, L., ed. 1998. *The power of servant leadership.* San Francisco: Berrett-KoehlerPublishers.

Wheatley, M., and M. Kellnor-Rogers. 1996. *A simpler way.* San Francisco: Berrett-Koehler Publishers.

Wood, S. 1995. Mountain climber urges nurses to gain strength from challenges. *National Teaching Institute's NTI News (American Association of Critical Care Nurses).* May15:1, 6.

Figure 5–1

EIGHT-POINT FRAMEWORK

(Kouzes and Posner 1993)

- Think first about your past

- Determine what you want

- Write an article about how you've made a difference

- Write a short vision statement

- Act on your intuition

- Test your assumptions

- Become a futurist

- Rehearse with visualizations and affirmations

NOTES

GENDER ISSUES IN LEADERSHIP | 6

INTRODUCTION

Androgyny signifies the blending of assertiveness, competitiveness, and dominance with concern for relationships, cooperativeness, and humanitarian values. It is necessary for men and women to be more androgynous whether they are leaders or followers. In all cases, most nurses need to practice being more team-oriented, less sensitive to criticism, and more focused on the present and future than on the past.

Perhaps the most significant step nurses could take in becoming more team-oriented would be to become involved in team learning, a concept that is different from team building. *Team building* focuses on communicating better within a team, and *team learning* focuses on learning and working collectively, the way, for example, that a winning sports team functions (Senge et al. 1994).

The point of team learning is to help people realize that the number of baskets or goals an *individual* makes is not nearly as important as how well the *entire* team plays. Indeed, it is the *total* number of baskets or goals a team generates that wins games. Perhaps with more women playing sports from an early age and more attention being focused on a work unit's productivity, nurses will be able to band together into a collective that uses each individual's strengths to create a group focus, rather than the individualistic focus with which so many of us are comfortable. The need to excel and be the best at something is a good trait, but not if it is exercised at the expense of the group or work unit.

As a whole, nurses can benefit from becoming more politically astute and more skilled at influencing others. Certainly nursing could gain in innumerable ways if the profession were to be more successful in influencing others! The arts of persuasion (being able to modify another's behavior or attitude) and negotiation (being able to resolve conflict in a way that is acceptable to both conflicting groups or individuals) are therefore necessary skills for women as well as men.

Nurses and women need to be increasingly visible, have autonomy in their ability to make decisions, feel that their contributions are necessary and relevant, and function as active members of working networks. No longer can they afford to be "out of the loop" or have their "heads in the sand." They can no longer be task-oriented and bury themselves in their personal work and goals; instead, they must be a part of team learning.

OBJECTIVES

- ♦ Analyze the unique qualities of feminine leadership.

- ♦ Describe the barriers that women face in exercising leadership in organizations.

- Propose strategies that women and men can use to enhance their effectiveness as leaders in organizations.

- Compare "web" organizations with "hierarchical" ones.

KEY WORDS

Androgyny	Negotiation	Team Building
Connective Leadership	Persuasion	Team Learning
Hierarchical Organizations	Politics	Web Organizations
Humanistic Leadership	Power	
Mentoring	Queen Bee Syndrome	

ACTIVITIES

1. Using Text Figure 6–2, "Becoming Androgynous," as a discussion topic, divide the class into mixed-gender small groups and ask them to give examples of the strategies listed. Be sure that men and women are working together on this assignment. Ask them to add any new ideas to the list, and caution them to avoid stereotypes.

2. Assign a short paper comparing Helgesen's (1990) web structure with Chaleff's (1995) idea of followers and leaders orbiting around a purpose rather than orbiting around a leader. (Text Chapter 3). To maximize this learning experience, have students discuss their thoughts after each student has prepared his/her own ideas.

3. Explore how a narrowing gender gap in nursing (i.e., with nurses become more androgynous) can be an advantage to the profession's political astuteness, power, flexibility and adaptability to change or develop new ideas, as well as its leadership position in healthcare. Point out the significance of nursing enjoying an "equal piece of the pie" in multidisciplinary meetings of teams that make major decisions about organizations. Have each student participate in a board meeting, such as an ethics committee; an ad hoc Panel; an interdepartmental meeting; or a church, local government, or university meeting. A one-page essay describing their observations of the roles assumed by three "major players" in the group — at least one of whom should be a woman — could be used to stimulate a discussion of gender similarities and differences in influencing group thinking. If attending such a meeting is difficult or impossible, have the students watch a televised meeting of the local school board or town council as a way to gather information for this assignment.

4. Have the students use Figure 6–1, "How to Measure Your Stress Level," to determine why they may not be able to concentrate on things other than their clinical practice or personal situation. Students may find it helpful to identify things that hinder them from focusing on broader issues and providing leadership. When women worry too much about their jobs, they become nonproductive in the rest of their lives. This exercise may show some individuals that it is up to them to do something about their stress. Of course, a dialogue with a mixed-gender group may facilitate growth.

5.   Have the students use Figure 6–2, "Political Self-Assessment Tool" (Goldwater and Zusy 1990), to determine how politically astute they are. Those with high scores could be asked to talk about what prompted them to take such an interest in the political arena and how they came to be so informed. Those with low scores could be asked to develop a plan and propose specific strategies that would increase their political astuteness. This tool could also be used as a way to measure the effect of the course on students' political awareness from the first to the last class session.

REFERENCES

Chaleff, I. 1995. *The courageous follower. Standing up to and for our leaders*. San Francisco: Berrett-Koehler Publishers.

Goldwater, M., and M. Zusy. 1990. *Prescription for nurses: Effective political action*. St. Louis: Mosby.

Helgesen, S. 1990. *The female advantage: Women's ways of leadership*. New York: Doubleday Currency.

How to measure your stress level. 1986. *Nursing Life* (May/June):46.

Senge, P., A. Kleiner, C. Roberts, R. Ross, and B. Smith. 1994. *The fifth discipline fieldbook*. New York: Doubleday.

Figure 6–1

HOW TO MEASURE YOUR STRESS LEVEL

(*Nursing Life* 1986)

To measure your own stress level during the past 24 hours, take this easy test. In a survey, staff nurses rated the 20 events listed here as "most stressful." Each of the events has an assigned stress value. Check the events you've experienced in the past 24 hours and then total their stress values. After you've taken the test, read below how to interpret the scores.

Stressful Work Event	Experienced? (Check if YES)	Stress Value
Assuming responsibilities you aren't prepared to handle	_____	67
Working with unqualified personnel	_____	64
Dealing with nonsupportive managers or administrators	_____	61
Working with insufficient staff	_____	58
Caring for a patient who's having a cardiac arrest	_____	55
Experiencing conflict with coworkers	_____	52
Dealing with a dying patient's family	_____	49
Caring for a dying patient	_____	46
Working with broken or faulty equipment	_____	44
Working with inadequate supplies	_____	42
Working an inconvenient shift or schedule	_____	38
Assuming responsibilities without getting thanks or recognition	_____	36
Dealing with a difficult doctor	_____	34
Trying to communicate with the hospital's bureaucracy	_____	31
Discharging a patient unprepared for discharge	_____	28
Caring for a seriously ill patient	_____	25
Spending long periods of time on paperwork or telephone duties	_____	22

Having a problem over salary or promotion	_____	19
Working with a demanding or noncompliant patient	_____	16
Coordinating supplemental personnel	_____	13

Interpretation of Scores

The higher the score, the more stress you've experienced in the past 24 hours. Estimate your present stress level by comparing your score with these:

0–133:   You are under minimal stress, but not enough to cause you many problems.

134–266:   You are under moderate stress. This is the highest level of stress that you should permit on a day-to-day basis.

267–532:   You are experiencing high-level stress. You have trouble relaxing, and you easily become annoyed. Try some stress-relieving exercises or enroll in a stress management course.

Figure 6–2

POLITICAL SELF-ASSESSMENT TOOL

(Goldwater and Zusy 1990)

Place a check next to those items for which the answer is "yes." Then give yourself one point for each "yes." After completing the inventory, compare your total score with the scoring criteria.

_____ 1. I am registered to vote.

_____ 2. I know where my voting precinct is located.

_____ 3. I voted in the last general election.

_____ 4. I voted in the past two elections.

_____ 5. I recognized the names of the majority of candidates on the ballot and was acquainted with the majority of issues in the last election.

_____ 6. I stay abreast of current health issues.

_____ 7. I belong to the state professional or student organization.

_____ 8. I participate (as a committee member, officer, etc.) in this organization.

_____ 9. I attended the most recent meeting of my district nurses' association.

_____ 10. I attended the last state or national convention held by my organization.

_____ 11. I am aware of at least two issues discussed and stands taken at this convention.

_____ 12. I read literature published by my state's nurses' association, a professional magazine, or other literature on a regular basis to stay abreast of current health issues.

_____ 13. I know the names of my senators in Washington, D.C.

_____ 14. I know the names of my representative in Washington, D.C.

_____ 15. I know the name of the state senator from my district.

_____ 16. I know the name of the representative from my district.

_____ 17. I am acquainted with the voting record of at least one of the above in relation to a specific health issue.

_____ 18. I am aware of the stand taken by at least one of the above in relation to a specific health issue.

_____ 19. I know whom to contact for information about health-related issues at the state or federal level.

_____ 20. I know whether my professional organization employs lobbyists at the state or federal level.

_____ 21. I know how to contact these lobbyists.

_____ 22. I contribute financially to my state and national professional organization's political action committee (PAC).

_____ 23. I give information about effectiveness of elected officials to assist the PAC's endorsement process.

_____ 24. I actively supported a senator or representative during the last election.

_____ 25. I have written to one of my state or national representatives in the past year regarding a health issue.

_____ 26. I am personally acquainted with a senator or representative or a member of his/her staff.

_____ 27. I serve as a resource person for one of my representatives or his/her aide.

_____ 28. I know the process by which a bill is introduced in my state legislature.

_____ 29. I know which senators or representatives are supportive of nursing.

_____ 30. I know which House and Senate committees usually deal with health-related issues.

_____ 31. I know the committees of which my representatives are members.

_____ 32. I know of at least two issues related to my profession that are currently under discussion.

_____ 33. I know of at least two health-related issues that are currently under discussion at the state or national level.

_____ 34. I am aware of the composition of the state board, which regulates the practice of my profession.

_____ 35. I know the process whereby one becomes a member of the state board, which regulates my profession.

_____ 36. I know what DHHS stands for.

_____ 37. I have at least a vague notion of the purpose of DHHS.

_____ 38. I am a member of a health board or an advisory group to a health organization or agency.

_____ 39. I attend public hearings related to health issues.

_____ 40. I find myself more interested in political issues now than in the past.

Scoring

0–9	Totally unaware politically
10–19	Slightly aware of the implications of politics on nursing
20–29	Beginning political astuteness
30–40	Politically astute... Asset to nursing

CHAOS AND DISEQUILIBRIUM... INVIGORATING, CHALLENGING, AND GROWTH-PRODUCING

7

As we move from the Scientific Age to the New Leadership Age, nurses must incorporate a new perspective: one that acknowledges that chaos is good because it makes us evolve and grow. This, of course, is contrary to almost everything that new or inexperienced nurses have learned. When caring for very sick people who experience one crisis after another, our goal as nurses has remained consistent: stabilize the patient and avoid chaos.

It is not until we develop a sense of knowing through experience and intuition that we as experienced nurses can actually welcome a change in the patient's status. What had previously looked like deterioration in a patient may, indeed, be a compensatory mechanism or a potentially favorable response. Some nurses can sometimes anticipate potential changes and can prepare the patient so that these changes have a less negative effect.

So what, one might ask, does this have to do with leadership? Actually, it has everything to do with leadership because it involves self-confidence and risk-taking, just as leadership does. It is through our leadership (i.e., our vision, creativity, flexibility, adaptability, power, motivation, empowerment, communication skills, ability to take risks, and stewardship) in the midst of crisis and chaos that the profession of nursing will survive and reach heights that we may never have thought possible. If it were not for the dramatic changes in healthcare experienced in recent years, for example, nurses might have remained mere assistants to physicians, dependent on others to give us "orders" by which we would plan our work. We might have continued to do things in certain ways because "that is how we have always done it" (Review Text Figure 7–1, "Time to Teach the Elephant to Dance" [Belasco 1990]). Instead, those of us in the field of nursing now find ourselves preparing advanced practice nurses for independent and collaborative practice; we are functioning as active, equal members of healthcare teams.

Dealing effectively with change is a talent that every nurse must cultivate. Being adaptable and flexible, as well as being able to "think on one's feet," are necessary skills for nurses practicing in this ever-changing world. Healthcare agencies are in the midst of the biggest changes they have ever experienced: merging, downsizing and upsizing, affiliating, acquiring, or whatever word one wishes to insert that connotes change. Some of the restructuring has been successful, but most has been viewed as far from positive for consumers, professionals, and organizations. Perhaps these less-than-positive results are a consequence of inadequate time for the various stages of change to evolve, a vision that was not strong enough to guide the change process, lack of clearly articulated core values that consistently guide decision making, poor communication, or lack of knowledge of what to expect (Kotter 1998).

Having a framework to guide planned change — such as Lewin's (1951) stages of unfreezing, moving, and refreezing — is often thought to be helpful. However, in many instances, change seems to evolve on its own, without any help from us. Perhaps the best strategy when facing change and chaos is to be aware, to not be afraid, to venture out, to ask questions, and to be happy that one is not bound to or by the status quo.

OBJECTIVES

♦ Describe the process by which leaders and followers can thrive and grow despite the chaos of the healthcare system.

♦ Describe how chaos can propel individuals and organizations to accomplish goals.

♦ Analyze how nurse leaders can use the change process effectively in the realization of a vision.

♦ Formulate strategies that decrease resistance to change.

♦ Describe how the purposeful introduction of conflict can generate change.

EY WORDS

Adaptability	Flexibility	Scientific/Newtonian Age
Change	Healthcare Redesign	
Chaos	New Leadership/Science	

ACTIVITIES

1. Have the students get into small groups and role-play the scenario noted below. Each student should role-play the nurse manager and various staff members. After the role-play is completed, ask students to discuss their actions, using Lewin's (1951) change theory as a framework. Be sure to point out the fact that stages of change are merely categories to help us in our thinking and that people can go back and forth between stages. Have the students incorporate Text Figure 7–3, "Results of Nurse Managers' Rankings of Healthcare Executives' Behavior during Change," when they engage in the role-play exercise.

   The nurse manager of a 60–bed surgical unit has decided that given the number of new staff on her unit, it is unsafe not to have a charge nurse for every shift. Her proposed solution is to institute a change from having no charge position to having a charge position for every shift.

2. Discuss Text Table 7–1, "The Use of Teams." Divide the class into two teams, one that favors the conventional assumptions about teams and another that argues for the new perspective about teams. Give each team 20 minutes to develop its platform; then randomly choose four individuals from each group to present their team's platform and to debate the advantages and disadvantages of the conventional perspective and the new perspective.

3. Use Text Figure 7–4, "The Readiness Quotient," to measure each student's readiness to change. Then ask all students to complete the questionnaire for the organization in which they work or have clinical rotations. Have the students discuss the advantages of using a tool like "The Readiness Quotient" when implementing a change.

4. Divide the students into small groups. Using Porter-O'Grady's (1998) "Rules for Achieving Change in an Organization" (Figure 7–1), have each group discuss the following proposed change scenarios:

(a) Nurses on each unit need to be cross-trained to work independently on another unit. Nurses can choose the unit to which they will be cross-trained, or every unit could "buddy" with another unit where all staff from each unit would be cross-trained.

(b) All nurses in a sub-acute facility need to learn how to draw blood, insert intravenous lines, and conduct comprehensive assessments. The majority of nurses have no experience with these skills, and there is only one nurse practitioner in the facility who can teach them.

(c) The 650-bed hospital has 8-hour shifts on all its nursing units. As a result of a feasibility study and the request of most of the 75 nurses involved (all but 10 senior nurses supported the proposed change), the medical division has decided to implement 12-hour shifts.

(d) The local home care agency is merging with another agency. In order to move the change along, the original agency's staff members need to be taught a new documentation program, and the administrators want the newly merged agency to have a fully functioning documentation system in 5 working days. Due to Medicare and Medicaid regulations, there will be major financial ramifications if the documentation program is not successfully implemented in 5 days.

(e) The new CEO of the hospice was hired with the understanding that all staff would be professionals, with the exception of the maintenance and dietary departments. This agreement means that six nursing assistants from each of the eight units will have to be terminated.

(f) The administration has just mandated that every RN be assigned 12 to 18 hours of overtime per week until the staffing shortage is alleviated. The majority of staff is elated about the prospect of making additional money, but there are some nurses who are not able to accommodate this mandate.

5. Have the students share their opinions on Critical Thinking Exercise #3 in Text Chapter 7 ("Given the "State of the Art" of Nursing, Do We Need a Revolution?"). Discuss how a revolution could empower nurses and the profession.

REFERENCES

Belasco, J. 1990. *Teaching the elephant to dance: Empowering change in your organization.* New York: Crown Publishers.

Kotter, J. 1998. Leading change: Why transformation efforts fail. In *Harvard Business Review on change*, 1–20. Boston: Harvard Business School Publishing.

Porter-O'Grady, T. (1998) The seven basic rules for successful redesign. In E. C. Heim (Ed.), Contemporary leadership behavior: Selected readings (5th Ed.) pp. 226–235.

Figure 7–1

RULES FOR ACHIEVING CHANGE IN AN ORGANIZATION

(Porter-O'Grady 1998)

- No Exceptions

- Read the Signs

- Construct a Vision

- Empower the Center

- Construct New Architecture

- Always Have a Plan of Action

- Evaluate, Adjust, Evaluate Again

SHAPING A PREFERRED FUTURE FOR NURSING

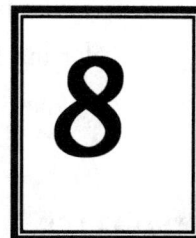

8

Leaders are responsible for articulating a preferred future for our profession and its practitioners, whether they be in clinical, administrative, educational, research, health policy, or other roles. Therefore, those of us in the profession have to make a concerted effort to increase the visibility of nurses, enhance the image of the profession, work together in validating nurses' contributions to providing effective and efficient patient care, develop partnerships, network with all members of the healthcare team, and promote increased access to nurses for all people in need of healthcare.

Nurses need to rally and work together to develop health policy that mandates quality healthcare for the uninsured, impoverished, and illiterate. These populations cannot be overlooked; they will continue to present massive problems for the world if they do not receive appropriate care and attention to health promotion for physical, psychological, social, and developmental growth. Substance abuse, teen pregnancy, increasing infant mortality, violence, and destruction of the family unit are increasing in every city as well as in many suburbs and rural towns. The time is here for all nurses to "tell their stories" about how they helped and how others can and must help so that the preferred future will be a reality for nurses and the people nurses serve. Nurses must educate the public on the importance of being proactive, not merely reactive.

Nurse leaders need to know a particular area well, understand how changes in this area began and have evolved, and be knowledgeable about how patterns of related happenings might impact that particular area currently and in the future. This kind of information will assist the leader in knowing how and where to study trends and in identifying indicators of future patterns.

OBJECTIVES

♦   Analyze how current societal healthcare trends can affect nursing's future.

♦   Examine projections for the future that are likely to affect the nursing profession and healthcare.

♦   Describe the characteristics of leaders who are needed to shape a preferred future for nursing.

♦   Formulate strategies that can prevent or minimize the potentially negative social, political, economic, and organizational forces that can affect the future of nursing.

♦   Suggest strategies whereby members of the nursing profession can create our own preferred future.

KEY WORDS

Empowerment	Possible Future	Quality Improvement
Nursing Taxonomy	Preferred Future	Vision
Plausible Future	Probable Future	

ACTIVITIES

1. Have the students discuss the meaning of the following statement about the negative aspect of managed care: *Healthcare is overmanaged and underled.* What can nursing leaders do to improve healthcare so that it is not overmanaged and underled?

2. Review Kouzes and Posner's (1995) survey, which asked leaders what they identify as significant to vision building (e.g., foresight, focus, forecasts, future scenarios, and perspectives). Ask students to develop their personal vision that describes a preferred future for nursing.

3. Divide the class into small groups of three and four. Using Minkin's (1995) TIP Approach ("Trends, Implications, and Predictions"), have each group brainstorm about where they would like to see nursing proceed in the near and distant future. Prior to this class session, have each student bring in information (from the Internet, newspaper, or a journal) about future predictions or trends that are expected to have an impact on healthcare; incorporate this information into the discussion of nursing's future.

4. Contact your State Nurses Association and ask a member of the N-STAT team (the "grassroots" component of the American Nurses Association) to speak to your class about empowering nurses through legislative and political action. Have the students get involved in some aspect of assisting the N-STAT representative.

5. Using the right side of Text Figure 8–2, "Characteristics of the Past/Traditional and Future Healthcare Systems" (adapted from Buerhaus 1998), have the students analyze the ways in which current societal healthcare trends are likely to affect the nature of the future healthcare system. Identify what nurses can do to assist in this transformation. Discuss the changes recommended by the PEW Commission for Nursing (Figure 8–1) that can assist in developing a preferred future.

6. Review the leadership project topic ideas in Appendix D. Incorporate a leadership project (possibly allocating one course credit for it) on the topic of the students' choice. If the course does not allocate credit for a leadership project, students can propose such a project hypothetically and outline a plan needed for its success

7. Have students review the example of a CTICU nurse's work with using forced warm air blankets post-operatively (see Text Chapter 8). Ask each to identify a clinical practice problem, review the literature, determine relevant clinical findings, outline a plan to change practice related to the clinical problem based on documented findings, implement the change, and evaluate the ramifications of the change. Discuss the significant difference for the patients and the cost savings for the institution that this change could have. This learning exercise is a good example of how students can learn to shape practice and not merely respond to changes made by others.

Bennis, W. 1989. *On becoming a leader.* Reading, MA: Addision-Wesley

Buerhaus, P. 1998. *Creating a new place in a competitive market: The value of nursing care.* In *Contemporary leadership behavior: Selected readings.* 5th ed, 422–431). Edited by E. C. Hein. Philadelphia: Lippincott-Raven.

Donaho, B. 1997. *The PEW Commission Report: Nursing's Challenge to Address It.* ANA, 2, 507–514.

Kouzes, J., and B. Posner. 1995. *The leadership challenge: How to keep getting extraordinary things done in organizations.* 2d ed. San Francisco: Jossey-Bass.

Minkin, B. 1995. *Future in sight.* New York: MacMillan.

Valiga, T. 1994. Leadership for the future. *Holistic Nursing Practice* 9:83–90.

Figure 8–1

RECOMMENDATIONS BY THE PEW COMMISSION ON NURSING

(Donaho 1997)

- ♦ Standardize regulatory terms

- ♦ Standardize requirements for entry into practice

- ♦ Remove barriers to the full use of competent professionals

- ♦ Redesign the state board structure and function

- ♦ Inform the public

- ♦ Collect data on the workforce

- ♦ Ensure the competence of practitioners

- ♦ Reform the professional disciplinary process

- ♦ Evaluate regulatory effectiveness

- ♦ Understand the organizational context of health professions regulation

Donaho, B. 1997. *The PEW Commission Report: Nursing's Challenge to Address It.* ANA, 2, 507–514.

FOUR KINDS OF FUTURES

(Valiga, 1994)

- ◆ Probable Future

- ◆ Possible Future

- ◆ Plausible Future

- ◆ Preferred Future

SHAPING A PREFERRED FUTURE

(Bennis, 1989)

- ◆ Manage the dream

- ◆ Embrace error

- ◆ Encourage reflective back-talk

- ◆ Encourage dissent

- ◆ Possess the Nobel

- ◆ Understand the "Pygmalion Effect"

- ◆ Develop the "Gretzky Factor"

- ◆ See the long view

- ◆ Understand the stakeholder's symmetry

- ◆ Create strategic alliances and partnerships

SHAPING A PREFERRED FUTURE

(Kouzes & Posner,1995)

- Do not wait

- Have credibility

- Have your head in the clouds… but your feet on the ground

- Share values

- Accept that you cannot do it alone

- Remember that you cannot do it alone

- Remember that leadership is everyone's business

NOTES

LEADERSHIP DEVELOPMENT AS A LIFELONG TASK... SELF AND OTHERS

9

INTRODUCTION

Nurses must set a standard of excellence for themselves and accept responsibility for influencing change in healthcare. To accomplish these goals, nurses must gain self-confidence, a goal that can be achieved by becoming competent in creating new strategies to provide healthcare, participating in developing healthcare policy, and partnering with others. Nurses must learn to write grants, network with community agencies, share expertise and resources, prepare educational materials, and assist in implementing health policy. Preparation for a leadership role begins at the undergraduate level and continues throughout one's career; therefore, it is paramount that nurses continue to build teams, improve conflict resolution skills, enhance communication skills, facilitate participation in shared governance structures, collaborate, and improve mentoring skills.

OBJECTIVES

♦ Describe ways in which individuals can develop as leaders.

♦ Describe the characteristics of an environment that facilitates the development of leadership skills in self and others.

♦ Relate the concept of empowerment to the development of leaders.

♦ Analyze the process of mentoring as it relates to the development of leaders.

♦ Propose a personal plan for leadership development that attends to empowerment, mentoring, role modeling, networking, self-assessment, and continued renewal.

KEY WORDS

Authoring/Writing	Entrepreneurship	Nurturing
Career Advancement	Goal-Directed Action	Precepting
Career Path	Graduate Education	Presentation Skills
Career Satisfaction	Lifelong Learning	Role Modeling
Consulting	Mentoring	Trajectories/Timelines

ACTIVITIES

1. Assign the students the following "challenge." After all have had a chance to complete this assignment, use class time to read each other's introductions and discuss how each participant was able to become so accomplished.

   The year is 2020. You are the keynote speaker at a major professional conference being attended by 1000 nurses, physicians, social workers, and other healthcare professionals. The conference organizers have asked you to write your own introduction so that the audience will be well aware of all your professional accomplishments and the contributions you have made to nursing. Write that introduction so that it does not exceed one page. Now, the year is 2000. What do you need to plan to do throughout your career to ensure that the introduction in 2020 is not pure fantasy? How will you go about doing it?

2. Ask students to identify a nurse that they wish to interview. The nurse may be a clinical preceptor, a faculty member, an alumnus of the School of Nursing, the president of a nursing organization, etc. Students should use the following set of questions to explore with this nurse the extent to which she/he was guided/mentored by other nurses and the effect that had on her/his career. They should then relate this nurse's experiences to literature about mentoring.

   Did you have a mentor? How did the relationship begin? Did you seek out the mentor or did the mentor select you?

   What type of relationship did/do you have with your mentor?

   If you did not have a mentor, do you think your career would have had a different outcome?

   Do you currently mentor someone? How would you describe this relationship?

3. Assign the students the following "career orchestration" exercise. Then use class time to discuss the strategies each has designed.

   You have unlimited funds, unlimited time, and open access to anyone in the world. Design a strategy that would be most effective in helping you develop yourself as a leader. Be specific regarding the types of classes you would take, the workshops you would attend and/or the degrees you would pursue, the nature of any mentoring experiences you would want, the kind of involvement you would want in professional organizations or community boards, and any other activities in which you would want to participate. Provide rationale for each step in your proposed "plan of attack".

4. Ask students to diagram their professional networks: who introduced them to whom, how they got to know various people, who has what kind of expertise that might be used, etc. You may want to use your own career network as an example, or use the one provided here.

   Consultations Grant Writer & Project Director Nursing Executive in Magnet Hospital

   MSN at Prestigious University

   Speaking Engagements Students Leader Dean

5. Ask each student to interview three different nurses and think about the following questions:

    What factors do these nurses identify as making nursing a satisfying career? What patterns do the students see emerging from these interviews?

6. Then ask all students to talk to four other students in the class (as assigned) about the findings of their interviews and the patterns they saw emerge. Ask them to talk with one another about what seem to be the most significant factors in finding satisfaction in one's career as a nurse. Then ask the group to take these factors and prepare a description of the "ideal" scenario to promote career satisfaction for nurses. The groups must address what a basic educational program should be and what it should provide; the personal skills, values, and characteristics nurses would need to develop; what nurses could look for in an employment setting; and what the profession as a whole could do to promote career satisfaction.

REFERENCES

Sandler, B.R. (1993). Women as mentors: Myths and commandments (Opinion). *The Chronicle of Higher Education,39(27), B3.*

GENERAL APPROACHES
TO LEADERSHIP DEVELOPMENT

- ♦ Lecture and Discussion… Formal Courses
- ♦ Role Play and Simulation
- ♦ Sensitivity Training
- ♦ Role Modeling
- ♦ Institutes and Fellowships
- ♦ On-the-Job Training

SOURCES OF EMPOWERMENT

- Empowering Workplace

- Environment

- Someone with Power

- Being Held Accountable for One's Work

- Shared Governance Models

- Knowledge and Expertise in an Area

- Knowledge of Self… Self Confidence

- Control of Self Growth

- Active Participation… at Work, in One's Community, etc.

CHARACTERISTICS OF MENTORS

- Close, trusted, experienced Counselor

- Accomplished Individual

- Good Friend and "Good Parent"

- Able to Guide the Protégé through Significant Points in her/his Career

- Able to Provide Counsel during Stress and Risk-taking Endeavors

- Able to Teach the Protégé

- Inspires and Challenges the Protégé

MYTHS ABOUT MENTORS

(Sandler, 1993)

♦ The best way to succeed is to have a mentor

♦ Mentoring is always beneficial

♦ The mentor should be older than the protégé

♦ A person can have only one mentor at a time

♦ If you want to have a mentor, you have to wait to be asked

♦ Men are better mentors for women

♦ When a man mentors a woman, the chances are great that it will develop into a sexual encounter

♦ The mentor always knows best

CHARACTERISTICS ATTRACTING MENTORS
OR... WHAT A MENTOR
LOOKS FOR IN A PROTÉGÉ

- Intelligence

- A self-starter... Someone who is internally motivated

- Someone who is looking for new challenges

- Good interpersonal and communication skills

- A risk-taker

- A hard worker

- Someone who has and understands ideas

- Someone with integrity

Continued

CHARACTERISTICS ATTRACTING MENTORS OR ... WHAT A MENTOR LOOKS FOR IN A PROTÉGÉ

- Someone who presents her/himself professionally

- Someone with a sense of humor

- Someone who is willing to invest in her/himself

- Someone with a curious mind… who asks questions

- Someone who has a visions… for her/himself and for the profession

NOTES

76

CONCLUSIONS... THE NEW LEADERSHIP CHALLENGE, EXCELLENCE, AND PROFESSIONAL INVOLVEMENT

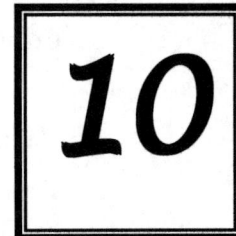

10

INTRODUCTION

As individuals take on the challenge of leadership and attempt to create a preferred future, they will encounter many who will assert that "things are not so bad," "we don't really need to change too much," and "the status quo is just fine". For those without the true passion that accompanies a vision, it may be quite appealing to "leave well enough alone."

However, those individuals who are committed — to a better practice environment, higher quality care for the poor and underserved, a greater emphasis on health promotion, stronger alliances between nursing practice and nursing education, more visible and influential roles for nurses in the health policy arena, or any number of other powerful visions — are unable to accept that they should "leave well enough alone." Instead, their passion for excellence drives them toward realization of their vision, and they employ a wide range of strategies to create the preferred future they envision.

Nurses with this drive for excellence are likely to be quite involved professionally, hold themselves and those with whom they work to the highest of standards, be willing to engage in confrontation to advance their cause, and take advantage of any opportunity to promote their view of a better world. They are likely to serve as mentors to neophytes in the profession, be thought of as the "movers and shakers" in the field, and be sought out for advice and counsel. In other words, they are seen as the leaders in nursing and the ones who will create the future we prefer.

OBJECTIVES

♦ Analyze the concept of excellence.

♦ Discuss the responsibility for promoting excellence held by leaders who will create nursing's preferred future.

♦ Examine the interrelations among leadership, excellence, and professional involvement.

♦ Propose strategies for exercising leadership, promoting excellence, and being professionally involved in order to create nursing's preferred future.

KEY WORDS

Accept the Challenge	Habits of Excellence	Preferred Future
Commitment	Mediocrity	Professional Involvement
Dreams	"Mirror Test"	Quality
Excellence	Passion	Status Quo
Flawlessness	Perfection	
"Get-it-all-together" Focus	Perseverance	

ACTIVITIES

1. After students have completed Critical Thinking Exercise #3 (see Text), use at least 1 hour to discuss what they gleaned from their interviews with nurses who recently received an award for excellence. Ask each student to share the two or three *most significant* things they learned from the interview. Record those items on the board, being sure to note points made by several students. When all students have shared their most significant insights, review the list with the class. Highlight those things that help develop a more definitive definition of the concept of excellence, particularly as it relates to nursing, and work in small groups (four to five students each) or with the class as a whole to formulate a definition of excellence in nursing. Then challenge students to use that definition as the "benchmark" against which to measure their own practice and performance as a student and to reflect on this in their course or clinical journal.

2. Review the criteria and procedures for selecting the Teacher or Nurse of the Year or the Most Outstanding Student in your nursing program or university. For each criterion, ask students to reflect on its meaning, how it could be "measured," and what "evidence" they would expect to see to determine whether an individual met it. Also ask them to reflect on the procedure for selecting the recipient of this honor and to discuss the basis for making such selections. Then discuss what excellence means in our culture and in other cultures throughout the world, how we know excellence when we see it, and how acknowledging true excellence is different from winning a "popularity contest". If such awards do not exist in your institution, have the students formulate a proposal to initiate one. They will need to consider what they mean by excellence in the area (i.e., teacher or student), develop criteria for selection, determine the kind of "evidence" that should be put forth to support a candidate for the award, and determine the procedure for selection. The same discussions can then occur.

3. Ask students to vote (via a written ballot that is kept confidential) for the one student in the class that they think best exemplifies excellence, leadership, *and* professional involvement. In order to be counted, a vote must be supported by rationale or examples in each of the three areas. Once all valid votes are tallied, discuss the outcomes (sharing names only if that seems appropriate), and, more importantly, discuss the rationale/support provided and the thinking in which the students engaged when casting their votes.

4. Ask all students to write a haiku about excellence, leadership, and professional involvement and submit it to you several days before the class session in which they will be discussed. Compile all poems into a single handout, using student author names if you think that would be appropriate for the group. Ask students to read the handout before class and be prepared to discuss the content

of the poems, the passions that are conveyed in them, and the extent to which these expressions are congruent with the literature about excellence and leadership.

5. Visit the following sites to learn more about selected professional organizations:

http://www.ana.org (American Nurses Association)

http://www.nln.org (National League for Nursing)

http://www. phikappaphi.org (Phi Kappa Phi)

http://www.nursingsociety.org (Sigma Theta Tau)

REFERENCES

Diers, D. and Evans, D. L. (1980). Excellence in nursing (Editorial). *Image, 12(2)*, 27–30.

Figure 10–1

COMPONENTS OF EXCELLENCE *

- Discipline

- Choreography

- Responsibility

- Caring

- Skepticism

- Perseverance

- Passion

Diers, D. and Evans, D. L. (1980). Excellence in nursing (Editorial). *Image, 12(2)*, 27–30.

ELEMENTS OF EXCELLENCE

- ◆ Strive to be the best we can be in everything we do

- ◆ Set high standards

- ◆ Do not accept mediocrity

- ◆ Do not accept the status quo

- ◆ Strive for perfection

- ◆ Challenge ourselves

- ◆ Seek out new experiences

- ◆ Maintain a broad perspective

- ◆ Go "above and beyond" what is required

- ◆ Pursue our passion

QUALITY

IS

NEVER

AN

ACCIDENT

EVERY JOB IS A SELF-PORTRAIT

AUTOGRAPH YOUR WORK WITH EXCELLENCE

EXCELLENCE
IS NOT
AN ISOLATED ACT,
BUT A HABIT.

EXCELLENCE

can be attained if you...

- ◆ CARE more than others think is wise,

- ◆ RISK more than others think is safe,

- ◆ DREAM more than others think is practical, and

- ◆ EXPECT more than others think is possible.

NOTES

Appendix A
Guidelines to and Evaluation of Class Participation

GUIDELINES TO CLASS PARTICIPATION

As evolving nurse leaders, students should develop skills of discussion, questioning, analysis, synthesis, and challenging others' ideas in a professional way. Participation in the classes for this course provides an opportunity to develop such skills.

During each class session, there will be an open discussion on a selected topic or several formal presentations made by faculty members, students, or guest speakers. The purposes of these open discussions and presentations are to provide information about selected concepts and to offer unique, creative perspectives on or ideas about those concepts.

As participants in these discussions or members of the "audience" for presentations, we should think and read about the topics in advance; formulate some of our own ideas and questions about them; and be prepared to discuss the topics in a thoughtful, scholarly way. In this way, class sessions become stimulating and challenging.

Prior to each discussion session or presentation, the entire class will receive information about the material to be addressed. Students are encouraged to seek out resources related to the topic. In addition, the instructor can provide relevant references, and all presenters should be able to do the same for those students who desire such assistance. All students are expected to read about the topics before each class.

Following each formal presentation, there will be a time-limited discussion period. During this time, class members will be expected to question, challenge, and/or offer comments to the presenter. These questions/comments should be thoughtful, reflective, and scholarly and should show that the "audience" is thinking about and analyzing what the presenter said as well as synthesizing the new ideas with those previously discussed in class sessions.

Each student will complete a self-evaluation regarding her/his class participation using the Class Participant's Self-Evaluation form. This form is to be completed at midterm and submitted to the instructor on the date specified. The instructor will review the form, add her comments, assign a grade for class participation up to that point, and return the form to the student. **Using the same form**, each student will complete this same process at the end of the semester. The student's class participation will be evaluated using the following criteria.

- ◆ Questions or comments relate clearly to the topic at hand.

- ◆ Questions are clearly and succinctly articulated.

- ◆ Questions reflect serious thought about the topic. They offer depth and are not merely superficial.

- ◆ Appropriate, relevant literature is cited.

♦ Comments help the class synthesize new ideas with those previously discussed.

♦ Questions are stimulating and challenging, encouraging others to respond with similar or dissimilar viewpoints.

♦ Comments and questions reflect unique perspectives or ideas on the topic.

♦ Comments are critical of ideas expressed in the presentation and/or in relevant literature.

♦ The student shows interest in the discussion and listens attentively.

♦ The student avoids dominating the discussion.

♦ The student participates actively in discussions in a consistent manner.

Developed by Theresa M. Valiga, EdD, RN

NAME: _____

CLASS PARTICIPANT'S SELF-EVALUATION

This tool should be used to facilitate your evaluation of your own contributions to class sessions and to document your progress in this area throughout the semester. Be objective as you rate yourself on the extent to which you think you achieved each of the following criteria, using the following scale: A = excellent, B = very good, C = average, D = poor, and F = not at all. Complete the columns on the left and page 2 at **midterm** and the columns on the right and page 3 at **the end of the course**. The midterm self-evaluation is to be submitted on **(Date)**, and the final self-evaluation is to be submitted on **(Date)**.

MIDTERM	CRITERION	FINAL
A B C D F	Raised questions/made comments that clearly related to the topic at hand	A B C D F
A B C D F	Posed questions clearly and succinctly	A B C D F
A B C D F	Made comments that reflected serious thought about the topic, offered depth, and were not superficial	A B C D F
A B C D F	Cited relevant literature appropriately	A B C D F
A B C D F	Made comments that helped the class synthesize new ideas with those previously discussed	A B C D F
A B C D F	Posed questions that were stimulating and challenging, encouraging others to respond with similar or dissimilar viewpoints	A B C D F
A B C D F	Made comments/posed questions that reflected unique perspectives or ideas on the topic	A B C D F
A B C D F	Made comments that were critical of ideas expressed in the presentation and/or in the literature	A B C D F
A B C D F	Showed interest in discussions and listened attentively	A B C D F
A B C D F	Avoided dominating discussions	A B C D F
A B C D F	Participated actively in discussions in a consistent manner	A B C D F

Generally, my **STRENGTHS** as a class participant at the midpoint of the semester are as follows:

Generally, the **AREAS I NEED TO STRENGTHEN** to be more effective as a class participant include the following:

Overall, the grade I think I earned for my participation in classes through the midpoint of the semester is as follows (circle one):

A+ A A- B+ B B- C+ C C-

INSTRUCTOR COMMENTS AND MIDTERM GRADE:

90

Overall, my **STRENGTHS** as a class participant throughout the semester were as follows:

Overall, the **AREAS I NEED TO STRENGTHEN** to be more effective as a class participant include the following:

Overall, the grade I think I earned for my participation in all classes throughout the semester is as follows (circle one):

A+ A A- B+ B B- C+ C C-

INSTRUCTOR COMMENTS AND FINAL GRADE:

Developed by Theresa M. Valiga, EdD, RN

Appendix B

Guidelines to and Evaluation of Leadership Project and Leader Analysis Options

LEADERSHIP PROJECT

The purpose of this project is to operationalize a leadership role as a professional nurse. The assignment is designed to allow the student to use the theory and skills learned in formal courses by developing, implementing, and evaluating a professional nursing activity that exemplifies leadership.

Upon completion of the Leadership Project, students will have:

♦ Completed all assigned forms correctly and completely.

♦ Submitted all assigned forms on the assigned dates.

♦ Documented a valid investment of the one (1) clinical credit (45 hours).

♦ Obtained necessary approvals before proceeding with the project.

♦ Presented a neatly typed report that follows the required format.

♦ Used references appropriately to substantiate rationale.

♦ Used the APA (American Psychological Association) writing style manual to guide the presentation of the report.

The final report must be submitted on or before (Date... near the end of the semester). Other due dates for interim aspects of the project are indicated in the directions.

The written report will be counted as 25% of the final course grade, and the oral report of the project to classmates and faculty will be counted as an additional 25% of the final course grade.

Directions for Developing and Implementing the Project

Students are free to work as individuals or in a group of no more than four.

The Initial Proposed Project Report (copy attached) is to be completed and submitted to the instructor in class by (Date... approximately 2 weeks into the semester).

When approval of the project has been given, the feasibility of the project must be established. Complete the Feasibility Report (copy attached), and submit it on (Date). This report provides descriptive statements and basic information about your project that should be included in your formal letter to the agency where you wish to do the project. Use university stationery for this letter. Students may not contact an agency or begin project implementation until the feasibility of the project has been established, reviewed, and approved by the instructor

Develop a mechanism or mechanisms for determining whether the project has met the stated purpose. Review these mechanisms with the instructor *before* implementing the project.

If the approved plan for implementation is or must be revised in any way prior to actual implementation of the project, this revision *must* be discussed with the instructor and *written approval* must be obtained.

The *Progress Report* (copy attached) is to be submitted on or before **(Date)**.

The final typed project report is to be submitted on or before **(Date... near the end of the semester)**.

Guidelines and Evaluation Parameters for the Project Report

Cover Sheet

> Title
>
> Name(s) of Student(s)
>
> Course Number and Title
>
> Date Submitted
>
> Preceptor or Sponsor for the Project
>
> Consultant(s) (if used)

Table of Contents

Project Objectives/Participant Objectives (10 points)

Project Purpose (5 points)

> Provide a brief statement on the rationale for the project and the nature of the problem that was addressed. Use appropriate references to develop the rationale.

Project Description (15 points)

> Concisely and clearly describe the following:
>
> > What healthcare issue was addressed through the project, documenting the importance of the issue (e.g., statistics) and using references.

What the project entailed (what was done; who was involved; and how they were involved in developing the project, obtaining permission for implementation of the project, or evaluating project outcomes).

In this section, you may want to refer the reader to your course journal/log, correspondence, or other sources.

Significance to Nursing (10 points)

Discuss how the project operationalized and exemplified professional nursing leadership in relation to the health care delivery system. References may be used here.

Application of Leadership/Organizational Theory (15 points)

Analyze the process of developing, implementing and evaluating the project in terms of leadership, organizational structure, power, conflict management, and change theories. Present this section analysis in a format or framework that facilitates the reader's ability to recognize the use of these theories in the analysis. Provide examples.

Analysis of Implementation (15 points)

Analyze your implementation process in terms of the decision-making and problem-solving processes used, your degree of assertiveness, and the quality of your communication skills. Identify conflicts and problems and how they were managed by addressing the following:

- The decisions that had to be made and the process that occurred

- The anticipated and unanticipated problems you encountered and how they were managed

- Your degree of assertiveness (or lack thereof) with peers and faculty agency personnel and how this affected the project assignment

- The stressors you encountered in developing, implementing and evaluating the project. What were they? What was their source? Were they managed well or mismanaged? What could have been done to prevent their occurrence or to have reduced them?

If everything went smoothly—you had no hold-ups or problems, no unusual stressors, no missed appointments, no disappointments—think about why the project was so successful and present an analysis of your success.

Evaluation (10 points)

Use your project objectives as the basis for reporting the findings of your evaluation. Provide a rationale for the mechanisms you selected to evaluate the outcomes of this project.

Bibliography (5 points)

Appendices

Copies of report forms

Copies of all correspondence

Log of the activities of each student involved in the project (5 points)

Copies of all relevant materials used

<u>Style, Grammar, Format, and Presentation (10 points)</u>

LEADERSHIP PROJECT

INITIAL PROPOSED PROJECT REPORT

Name(s) of student(s):_____

_____

_____

Date: _____

What do you propose to do for this project?

_____

_____

_____

Where will do you propose doing the project?

_____

Who do you hope will participate in this project (i.e., audience)?

_____

_____

What are your ideas about how you will recruit participants?

_____

_____

_____

How long do you think it will take you to prepare for the project?   _____

How many minutes/hours do you think it will take to actually do the project? _____

How did you determine these lengths of time?

_____

_____

Why do you think that your proposed project is appropriate for a nurse to conduct?

_____

_____

_____

_____

List your objectives for your project. Use the format of "Upon completion of this project..." Note that your objectives must be written in measurable, observable, behavioral terms and must be derived from your purpose for the project.

_____

_____

_____

_____

_____   _____

(Signature of Instructor, indicating approval)   (Date)

LEADERSHIP PROJECT

FEASIBILITY REPORT

Name(s): _____

Project title: _____

Who has been contacted regarding implementation of this project?

     Name: _____

     Title: _____

Agency: _____

How was the contact made (phone, letter, personal contact, etc.)? _____

Was verbal permission granted?   Yes _____   No _____

If "Yes," have you forwarded a confirming letter?   Yes _____ No _____

If "No," briefly explain the problem: _____

_____

Have you received a confirmation letter from the agency?   Yes _____   No _____

If "Yes," attach a copy of that letter to this form.

If "No," when do you expect this letter to arrive? _____

NOTE: When it arrives, please revise this form, attach a copy, and provide your project preceptor/sponsor with a copy of both documents.

If permission has been granted and a letter of confirmation received, please provide the following information:

The date you expect to begin project implementation: _____

    The specific site(s) where you will implement the project: _____

If you *do not have verbal permission* yet, describe the problems you have encountered in getting the project under way and make an appointment *immediately* with your project preceptor/sponsor to discuss the difficulties and strategies to use to move ahead with the project.

_____

_____   _____

(Signature of Instructor, indicating approval)   (Date)

LEADERSHIP PROJECT

PROGRESS REPORT

Has implementation of the project occurred?   Yes _____   No _____

If "Yes," on what date(s) did implementation occur?   _____

If "No" because the planned date for implementation has not yet occurred, on what date are you scheduled to implement the project?   _____

If "No" because the originally scheduled date was cancelled:

What was the original date for implementation?   _____

What is the new date for implementation?   _____

Briefly explain the reason for the change in date.   _____

_____

If "No" for other reasons, please explain.   _____

_____

Has the project been implemented as planned and approved by the instructor?

Yes _____ No _____

If "Yes," give a brief status report.   _____

_____

_____

If "No," briefly explain the nature of any changes in the project and the reasons for thosechanges.

_____

LEADERSHIP PROJECT

GUIDELINES FOR PRESENTATION

The purpose of this assignment is to provide students with an opportunity to develop skill in making an effective presentation to a professional group. All individual or group presenters are expected to do the following:

♦ Develop a framework for the presentation of the content about the project.

♦ Emphasize the most important/key points during the presentation (i.e., background, rationale, purpose, significance to nursing, implementation processes [or plans for implementation], and mechanisms for evaluating the effectiveness of the project).

♦ Organize the content so that the presentation is concise and coherent.

♦ Develop an effective closure for the presentation that summarizes the key points.

♦ Complete the presentation within the allotted time.

♦ Actively involve all members of the group in a discussion following the presentation.

LEADERSHIP PROJECT

EVALUATION OF PRESENTATION

		Points Earned	Potential Points	Comments
1.	Provided a framework for organization of the presentation.	_____	__(10)__	_____
2.	Presented key facts about the background/rationale for doing the project.	_____	__(10)__	_____
3.	Described the objectives of the project; specified participant objectives.	_____	__(10)__	_____
4.	Discussed how the project was implemented, using the project objectives.	_____	__(25)__	_____
5.	Described the mechanisms used to evaluate the outcomes of the project; related these to the project objectives.	_____	__10)__	_____
6.	Presented content in a logical and organized manner.	_____	__(5)__	_____
7.	Stayed within the allotted time frame.	_____	__(5)__	_____
8.	Used audiovisual materials effectively.	_____	__(10)__	_____
9.	Provided a summary of the presentation.	_____	__(5)__	_____
10.	Answered questions in an articulate manner.	_____	__(10)__	_____

GUIDELINES FOR COMPARISON OF

A NURSE AND A NON-NURSE LEADER

One of the ways to learn about and develop effective leadership abilities is to analyze the values and actions of individuals who are or have been recognized as leaders. By studying their styles, the way they interact(ed) with others, the nature of the situations in which they "rose above the crowd," and the ways in which they use(d) power, one can develop an understanding of why these individuals are considered to be leaders and how they have been able to influence others in achieving goals. This assignment provides the student with the opportunity to engage in such an analysis.

Students will conduct a thorough review of the literature that describes/defines leaders and leadership and critique those descriptions/definitions in terms of their usefulness. As a result of this critical analysis, students should offer their definitions and description of leaders and leadership and "defend" or "justify" those definitions and descriptions. Literature related to power, change, creativity, credibility, image, style, leader/follower interactions, conflict management, envisioning goals, affirming values, motivating others, managing, achieving a workable unity, serving as a symbol, explaining, representing a group externally, or renewing self and others is appropriate for review and "interpretation."

Armed with this foundation, students can look more carefully and critically at the selected leaders. Each student's selection of individuals for analysis is to be submitted to the instructor for approval on or before **(Date... approximately 3 weeks into the semester)**.

Each student will select a contemporary or historical figure outside the field of nursing who is thought to be a leader. After reading works by or about the leader (and interviewing him/her, if possible), the student will write an analysis of that individual as a leader, using all elements of the definition/description of leaders and leadership she/he developed as a guide. Evidence should be provided from sources by or about the leader to support the student's conclusions about her/his leadership.

In an attempt to better understand our own discipline and to address the criticisms that "there are no leaders in nursing today," each student will also select a person in contemporary nursing whom she/he considers to be a leader and conduct a similar analysis of that individual. Again, references by or about the selected nursing leader as well as data gathered through a review of her/his curriculum vitae or an interview with her/him (if possible) should be used as the basis for the analysis. Such data should be used as evidence to support the student's conclusions about the nurse leader's leadership effectiveness.

After thoroughly analyzing the selected nurse and non-nurse leaders, the student will compare the two individuals as leaders. Conclusions about their effectiveness as leaders should be drawn.

Finally, the student will engage in a critical self-analysis of her/himself as a potential leader in nursing. Using the conclusions that were drawn about the selected individuals' effectiveness as leaders, the student should (1) examine her/his own strengths to exert effective leadership in the way the selected leaders did, (2) identify areas that need to be developed to assume an effective leadership role, and (3) formulate specific strategies to strengthen her/his leadership assets and develop her/his perceived limitations as a leader.

There is no limit to the length of this paper. It is to be submitted to the instructor on or before **(Date... at the end of the semester)** and will be evaluated using the following criteria.

- The review of literature is thorough and comprehensive.

- The critiques of published definitions and descriptions of leaders and leadership are thoughtful and relevant.

- The justification for the proposed definitions and descriptions of leaders and leadership is sound.

- The developed definitions and descriptions of leaders and leadership used to guide the analysis are articulated clearly and reflect attention to the limitations noted in existing definitions and descriptions.

- The analysis of the non-nursing leader is thorough and clearly articulated.

- The analysis of the non-nursing leader is done in relation to the developed definitions and descriptions of leaders and leadership.d

- Evidence is provided to support conclusions about the non-nursing leader's leadership.

- The analysis of the nursing leader is thorough and clearly articulated.

- The analysis of the nursing leader is done in relation to the definitions and descriptions of leaders and leadership developed.

- Evidence is provided to support conclusions about the nursing leader's leadership.

- The comparison of the two individuals as leaders evolves from the data provided in the analyses, is objective, is comprehensive, and clearly articulates the two individuals' similarities and differences as leaders.

- Conclusions drawn about the effectiveness of the two individuals as leaders are valid in light of the analyses and comparisons provided.

- The self-analysis is critical, examines personal strengths necessary to exert effective leadership, identifies areas that need to be developed to assume an effective leadership role, and proposes specific strategies to strengthen personal leadership assets and develop perceived limitations as a leader.

- Ideas from the literature are synthesized with the student's own ideas.

- Ideas throughout the paper are developed logically and succinctly.

- The paper is a scholarly product and reflects proper format (e.g., grammar, citation format, etc.).

The following resources may be helpful in selecting a nursing leader to analyze or in beginning to gather some information about the leader selected.

Blumberg, A., ed. 1995. *Great leaders, great tyrants?* Westport, CT: Greenwood Press.

Clark, L., and J. Quinn. 1987. A brave new world for nurses. *Nursing & Health Care*. 8: 7–13.

Felder, D. G. 1996. *The 100 most influential women of all time: A ranking past and present*. New York: Citadel Press.

Safier, G. 1977. *Contemporary American leaders in nursing: An oral history*. New York: McGraw-Hill.

Schorr, T. M., and A. Zimmerman. 1988. *Making choices, taking chances: Nurse leaders tell their stories*. St. Louis: Mosby.

Sharp, N. J. 1997. *The nurses' directory of capitol connections*. 4th ed. Bethesda, MD: Sharp Legislative Resources.

Developed by Theresa M. Valiga, EdD, RN

EVALUATION OF COMPARISON OF

A NURSE AND A NON-NURSE LEADER

The *Comparison of a Nurse and a Non-Nurse Leader* paper has been evaluated as follows, using the prespecified criteria. **A = excellent**, **B = very good**, **C = average**, **D = poor**, and **F = not at all**.

The review of literature was thorough and comprehensive.	A B C D F
The critiques of published definitions and descriptions of leaders and leadership were thoughtful and relevant.	A B C D F
The justification for the proposed definitions and descriptions of leaders and leadership was sound.	A B C D F
The developed definitions and descriptions of leaders and leadership used to guide the analysis were articulated clearly and reflected attention to the limitations noted in existing definitions and descriptions.	A B C D F
The analysis of the non-nursing leader was thorough and clearly articulated.	A B C D F
The analysis of the non-nursing leader was done in relation to the developed definitions and descriptions of leaders and leadership.	A B C D F
Evidence was provided to support conclusions about the non-nursing leader's leadership.	A B C D F
The analysis of the nursing leader was thorough and clearly articulated.	A B C D F
The analysis of the nursing leader was done in relation to the developed definitions and descriptions of leaders and leadership.	A B C D F
Evidence was provided to support conclusions about the nursing leader's leadership.	A B C D F

The comparison of the two individuals as leaders:

evolved from the data provided in the analysis	A B C D F
was objective	A B C D F
was comprehensive	A B C D F
clearly articulated the two individuals' similarities and differences as leaders.	A B C D F
Conclusions drawn about the effectiveness of the two individuals as leaders were valid in light of the analyses and comparisons provided.	A B C D F

The self-analysis:

was critical   A B C D F

examined personal strengths necessary to exert effective leadership   A B C D F

identified areas that need to be developed to assume an effective leadership A B C D F
role

proposed specific strategies to strengthen personal leadership assets and A B C D F
develop perceived limitations as a leader.

Ideas from the literature were synthesized with own ideas.   A B C D F

Ideas throughout the paper were developed logically and succinctly.   A B C D F

The paper was a scholarly product and reflected proper format (e.g., grammar, A B C D F
citation format, etc).

OVERALL COMMENTS AND GRADE:

Developed by Theresa M. Valiga, EdD, RN

Appendix C

Annotated Bibliography

Adams, R. 1972. *Watership Down.* **New York: Avon Books.**

Watership Down is a book about the adventures of a group of rabbits that leave their comfortable warren in search of a better, safer place to live. Originally thought of as a children's story, this book is an excellent portrayal of leadership styles, leader/follower interactions, and the qualities of effective leaders and followers.

The group of rabbits that serves as the focal point of the story travels extensively to reach its goal and encounters several different warrens along the way. The rabbits experience warrens that are leaderless and warrens that are headed by a totalitarian despot. They also discover warrens in which the "leader" provides direction and the basic needs of rabbits in the warren are met; in these warrens, however, there is an aloofness between the leader and followers, and high-order needs are not met.

The Watership Down rabbits form a democratic, participating group. In this group, the talents of each rabbit are known and called upon as needed, followers assume the role of leader when circumstances require a particular type of leadership, and there is a constant exchange of ideas and support. In essence, this group of rabbits exhibits all that is good about leaders and followers.

This book exposes the reader to various types of leadership and leader/follower relationships. One sees risk-taking, acting in uncertainty, clarity of vision, clear communication, and many other behaviors of leaders, all within the context of a beautiful story that captures the imagination and holds the attention.

Bass, B. 1985. *Leadership and performance beyond expectations.* **New York: The Free Press.**

This outstanding book describes leadership in terms of transformational and transactional components. The author says that transformational leadership is found in varying amounts in everyone and needs to be tapped. He offers traditional leaders, such as Moses, Buddha, Jesus Christ, and Mohammed, as well as contemporary leaders, such as Theodore Roosevelt, John F. Kennedy, and Gandhi, as examples for study. He also cites ways in which each of these individuals depicted charisma, individualized consideration, and intellectual stimulation. Bass also gives behavioral examples of transactional leadership and defines the principles of management-by-exception and contingent rewards.

Perhaps the most interesting aspect of this book is the description of the data collected from the author's classic study of 104 military officers who completed the author-developed Leadership Questionnaire, which asked the officers about their perceptions of their immediate supervisor's leadership skills. The findings — what these individuals believed made someone an effective leader — are extremely interesting. The results of this study also point out how an effective leader can influence the followers in a group. A copy of the Leadership Questionnaire and parameters for scoring are included.

Bass, B. M. 1990. *Bass and Stogdill's handbook of leadership: Theory, research, and management applications*. 3d ed. New York: The Free Press.

This is a classic volume that provides a historical perspective on leadership, an analysis of the meaning of leadership, descriptions of various categories or types of leadership, and an examination of leadership theories and models (including Great Man, trait, situational, psychoanalytic, and other theories). Beyond this introductory material, this 1000+-page book emphasizes research on leaders and leadership.

The reported research focuses on leadership traits, tasks of leaders, leadership styles, women and leadership, leader/follower interactions, and the significance of values to leaders. Such concepts as charisma, inspirational leadership, power, and conflict are also addressed.

This handbook is an excellent resource for any serious student of leadership. Sadly, the book has not been updated since 1990, so current research about leadership is noticeably absent. In addition, although the author notes that leadership and management are different phenomena, most of the studies reported use managers as subjects, thereby suggesting that one needs to be in a position of authority to be considered a leader. Despite these limitations, *Bass and Stogdill's Handbook of Leadership* is a classic that should be read and used as a reference source.

Beatty, J. 1998. *The world according to Peter Drucker*. New York: The Free Press.

This book chronicles the life of Peter Drucker and delineates how he constantly pushed himself to become a stronger and more successful person by thinking about what people can do, not only what they cannot do. Drucker is a firm believer of frequent self-evaluation, which he called "keeping score on self" (p. 14). This theme is inherent in all of his work.

Drucker is perhaps best known for his philosophy on "management by objectives," which emphasizes the significance of planning, setting goals, and evaluating results against pre-established expectations. All of this is clearly part of management, but it is also a crucial part of being an effective leader... namely, having a vision and evaluating, on a regular basis, the progress made toward realizing the vision.

This book is easy to read and gives the reader a feeling that one can be whatever one wants to be. It also stresses the importance of making a difference in people's lives and not being remembered merely for writing a book or developing a theory. This book is a good tool for helping individuals develop their leadership abilities.

Bennis, W. 1989. *On becoming a leader*. Reading, MA: Addison-Wesley.

Written by one of the foremost authorities on leadership, this book is a classic in the field. Beginning with the conviction that "each of us contains the capacity for leadership" (p. 3), the author leads the reader in a thoughtful, reflective exploration of the nature of this elusive phenomenon and the qualities and characteristics of those who serve as leaders.

Although leadership can be provided by almost anyone, leaders are not ordinary people, according to Bennis. They "work out there on the frontier (p. 5), they serve as "anchors in our lives" (p. 15), they take risks and fail but always learn from those failures, they engage in continuous learning and self-development, and they know themselves. Indeed, the author notes that leadership is a journey of personal development.

By using many examples — from Norman Lear to Gloria Steinem, from the executive director of the American Association of University Women to the chairman and CEO of Johnson & Johnson — Bennis helps the reader understand how leaders need to master the contexts in which they find themselves (and, indeed, create new contexts), use their instincts and intuition, and be innovators who help others move through chaos. These examples are also used to illustrate the differences between leadership and management.

Serious students of leadership will want this classic reference in their collection. It is insightful and offers many practical suggestions for developing as a leader.

Bennis, W., and B. Nanus. 1985. *Leaders. The strategies for taking charge*. New York: Harper & Row.

In this seminal work, the claim that "managers are people who do things right and leaders are people who do the right things" (p. 21) is first made. The authors discuss the dramatic changes taking place in our world and acknowledge the need for competent leadership and for "great flexibility and awareness on the part of leaders and followers alike" (p. 14).

Based on the results of a 2-year study of individuals who were considered leaders, Bennis and Nanus identified "four major themes/areas of competency/human handling skills" (p. 26) (; Where does this quote begin?) that emerged. Those strategies are attention through vision (i.e., creating a focus or having an agenda, particularly one that draws others in), meaning through communication (i.e., expressing ideas powerfully so that others understand and want to support them), trust through positioning (e.g., making one's position known, being reliable, and being "tirelessly persistent [with] relentless dedication" [p. 45]), and the deployment of self (i.e., having a positive self-regard, knowing one's strengths and weaknesses, and setting high goals). Each of these strategies is discussed thoroughly, and many ideas on implementation are offered.

The authors conclude by saying that "we must raise the search for new leadership to a national priority" (pp. 228–229). They urge the purposeful and continuous development of leaders because without effective leaders, the best our society can do is maintain the status quo; at worst, it could disintegrate.

Burns, J. M. 1978. *Leadership*. New York: Harper Torchbooks.

This book is truly a classic. It was Burns who first acknowledged that "leadership is one of the most observed and least understood phenomenon on earth" (p. 2) and then proceeded to help us understand this complex concept.

He notes the lack of knowledge about leadership and how to develop it — despite the hundreds of definitions of the term — and the negligible attention was given to the significance of followers and the "interwoven texture of leadership and followership" (pp. 4–5). He also analyzes the nature of power and the role of power in leadership and explores the ways in which leaders help release the potential of others.

In his attempt to clarify the meaning of leadership, Burns offers distinctions between *transactional* and *transformational* leadership and introduces the notion of *moral* leadership. In recent years, many authors have "carried the banner" of transformational leadership, but Burns was the first to name it and describe it exquisitely.

As a result of Burns's seminal work on leadership, our understanding of this complicated concept progressed enormously. This is a book that must be read as a foundation to subsequent works about leadership.

Chaleff, I. 1998. *The courageous follower: Standing up to and for our leaders.* **San Francisco: Berrett-Koehler Publishers.**

This book gets to the heart of what leadership truly is and how it grows from followership. The author describes followership in a very positive way and avoids the negative connotations often associated with being a follower.

Chaleff discusses being an *effective* follower; this, he says, makes all of the difference in generating effective leadership. He offers many fundamental, commonsense, helpful ideas that could be useful to the person interested in empowering herself or himself and others, creating a vision, making a change, and preparing for a leadership role.

The author makes a point of explaining the significance of being a follower, supporting the leader's vision, and participating actively in change processes. One major point is that followers do not do things simply at the bidding of leaders, nor do they hide behind leaders. Instead, followers do things because they think they are best for themselves and for the organization. Followers, according to Chaleff, are not weak or passive. They are dynamic and passionate about many issues.

This book is a "must read" for persons who wish to understand the relationship between leaders and followers and appreciate the significance of followers in making change and realizing visions.

Conger, J. 1992. *Learning to lead: The art of transforming managers into leaders.* **San Francisco: Jossey-Bass.**

Conger firmly believes that leadership can be "broken down" into specific behaviors and that those behaviors can be taught and learned. In fact, this book is an account of his own experiences in learning to be a leader through his participation in the following innovative leadership development programs: (a) Kouzes and Posner's Leadership Challenge, (b) the Center for Creative Leadership's Leadership Development Program, (c) the Experiential Pecos River Learning Center Program, and (d) the Vision Quest Program.

The author explains the significance of leaders having a vision, being inspirational, demonstrating charisma, being empowered, and acting as a transformational change agent. He asserts that one can learn these skills.

Conger identifies work experiences, unexpected opportunities, educational advancement, experiences with mentors, and hardship as variables that foster leadership. He explains the historical development of leadership training and points out the importance of having such programs focus on providing feedback to participants regarding their conceptual development, skill building, and personal growth.

Conger also explores some of the more "common" theories about leadership. He explains how situational leadership and the "task-versus-relationship" contingency model of the 1980s lack the strategic envisioning, inspirational speaking, and change managing that he feels are absolutely essential for an effective leader in today's environments. He believes that all aspiring leaders need to participate in the kind of personal growth programs that he discusses in this book.

Covey, S. 1991. *Principle-centered leadership.* **New York: Summit Books.**

This book is grounded in the idea that one's life can be more productive and fulfilling if one has principles to guide it . Covey presents his ideas about the principles of vision, leadership, and human relationships as the way to make decisions in one's personal, interpersonal, managerial, and organizational lives. He offers suggestions on how to cultivate eight characteristics that facilitate the making of what he calls a "principle-centered leader."

This excellent book on self-leadership can be used as a rich resource to assist others in their development as leaders, particularly "principle-centered" leaders. Covey's ideas center around the importance of a leader being a pathfinder — someone who can align an organization's or an individual's structure through an individual's behavior, *not* through the organization's behavior — and a facilitator or empowerer of others. To Covey, being a pathfinder means being able to move an individual or group down a path or allow it to accomplish its vision. The pathfinder is an individual who, by using leadership, moves someone or an organization in a new direction. This principle differs those that involve an organization's behavior, which dictate that more people change because they must live up to the organization's policies and expectations.

DePree, M. 1989. *Leadership is an art.* **New York: Currency Doubleday.**

This book is about "the art of leadership; liberating people to do what is required of them in the most effective and humane way possible" (p. 1). As an art, leadership is something one learns over time.

One of the most significant aspects of leadership, according to DePree, is a genuine concern for and about others. Leaders understand the diversity of the talents, gifts, and skills others possess and find ways to allow each individual to contribute to a cause or purpose in her/his way.

The author asserts that leaders serve others: "They are stewards more than they are owners... and they should leave behind them assets and a legacy" (p. 13). They are responsible for identifying, developing, and nurturing future leaders, and they bind people together to accomplish great things. They provide and help to maintain the momentum of a group, and they keep the group focused on the values and visions that guide them.

This easy-to-read book includes many insightful points about leaders and leadership that stimulate one's thinking in new ways. The conceptualization of leadership is an art, but an art that can be learned; it is useful for the would-be leader.

Dreher, D. 1996. *The Tao of personal leadership.* **New York: Harper Business.**

This book is a rich blend of the principle of centering and balancing one's life and the Taoist philosophy of simultaneously engaging in compassion and detachment. It emphasizes the importance of realizing the power of living systems that are generating energy all around us, and it reinforces the appreciation of all people potentially becoming leaders, regardless of their "station" in life.

Communication, team building, having an appetite for constant change, credibility, risk-taking, and the ability to help others accomplish goals and visions are necessary assets of a strong leader. The author describes the Tao leader as being a pioneer; a pathfinder; a person who guides with intuition; someone who constantly faces the unknown with excitement; and someone who turns conflict into opportunities for stronger relationships, greater knowledge, and better solutions. The author has written an exhilarating account of how one can develop one's leadership capacity in exponential fashion.

Gardner, J. W. 1990. *On leadership*. **New York: The Free Press.**

John Gardner is an expert on leadership. In this book, he reportsinsights gained from a 5-year study of the phenomenon. He distinguishes leadership from management and expresses the great need we have for true leaders, individuals "who are exemplary, who inspire, who stand for something, [and] who help us set and achieve goals" (p. xi).

One of the most significant contributions Gardner makes through this book is helping the reader understand what he calls "the tasks of leadership" Included in those "tasks" are the following:

- ◆ Envisioning Goals... pointing us in the right direction or asserting a vision

- ◆ Affirming Values... reminding the group of the norms and expectations they share

- ◆ Motivation... stimulating and encouraging others to act

- ◆ Managing... planning, setting priorities, and making decisions

- ◆ Achieving Workable Unity... managing conflict and promoting unity within the group

- ◆ Explaining... teaching followers and helping them understand why they are being asked to do certain things

- ◆ Serving as a Symbol... acting in ways that convey the values of the group and its goals

- ◆ Representing the Group... speaking on behalf of the group

- ◆ Renewing... bringing members of the group to new levels

In fulfilling these tasks, leaders must work collaboratively with followers, whom Gardner refers to as "constituents." He acknowledges that "followers often perform leader-like acts" (p. 23) and recognizes the significant role that followers play in accomplishing change and realizing vision.

Finally, Gardner draws on the work of many researchers to identify several attributes of leaders: physical vitality and stamina (i.e., a high energy level), intelligence and judgment-in-action (i.e., ability to identify and solve problems and set priorities), willingness to accept responsibilities (i.e., exercise initiative, bear the burden of making a decision, and step forward when no one else will), task competence (i.e., knowing the task at hand and the system), understanding of followers/constituents and their needs, skill in dealing with people, a need to achieve, the capacity to motivate others, and courage, among others. He also discusses how leaders need to use power and how they need to be morally responsible.

Greenleaf, R. 1998. *The power of servant leadership: Essays by Robert Greenleaf.* **Edited by L. Spears. San Francisco: Berrett-Koehler Publishers.**

This book captures the vision and writings of the late Robert K. Greenleaf, who was the first to use the term "servant leadership." According to Greenleaf, "servant leadership" is a way of leading that puts serving others (e.g., customers, patients, employees) first. This collection includes the following eight essays written by Greenleaf throughout his career: "Servant-Leadership: Retrospect and Prospect," "Education and Maturity," "The Leadership Crisis," "Have You a Dream Deferred?," "The Servant as Religious Leader," "Seminary as Servant," "My Debt to E. B. White," and "Old Age: The Ultimate Test of Spirit."

All of the essays in this collection reflect Greenleaf's ideas about spirit, commitment to vision, and wholeness. Given this focus, this is a most reflective book that leaves the reader with a feeling of "wanting to do things right."

***Harvard business review on leadership.* 1998. Cambridge, MA: Harvard Business School Press.**

These eight articles are written by some of the foremost thinkers in the area of leadership, namely Mintzberg, Kotter, Zaleznik, Badaracco, Heifetz, Laurie, Farkas, Wetlaufer, Teal, Berkley, and Nohria. Many of the articles have an executive summary proceeding them, and most are followed with a retrospective commentary by the author. Mintzberg, for example, even offers some self-study questions after his chapter.

These writings are significant because they raise key questions, such as the following: Are managers and leaders different? What do leaders really do? How do chief executives really lead? Why is providing leadership difficult?

At the end of the text, a short paragraph describes each of the contributing authors and their accomplishments since their seminal pieces were originally published. This book is definitely a required read.

Hein, E. C. ed. 1998. *Contemporary leadership behavior: Selected readings.* **5th ed. Philadelphia: Lippincott-Raven.**

This book is a collection of articles that were originally published in various journals. The articles are organized into categories that focus on the culture of nursing (e.g., caring and gender socialization), theories of leadership and attributes of leaders, leadership behaviors (e.g., assertiveness, advocacy, and mentoring), the organizational setting, and shaping nursing's future.

This is a good resource of varied articles and differing perspectives on topics relevant to leadership. Chapters can be read out of sequence, and no chapter depends on the preceding; therefore, readers have a great deal of flexibility in how to use the book.

Note: Previous editions of this book are also helpful references. The publication dates of those editions are as follows: 1st edition, 1982; 2nd edition, 1986; 3rd edition, 1990; and 4th edition, 1994. E.C. Hein and M.J. Nicholson edited the first three editions. Hein edited the 4th Edition.

Helgesen, S. 1990. *The female advantage: Women's ways of leadership.* **New York: Doubleday Currency.**

In this book, one of the few that deals specifically with women as leaders, Helgesen describes ways in which women lead differently than men. When studying women leaders in the workplace, she found patterns of behavior and approaches to making decisions and setting priorities that were quite different from what had been reported in studies of male leaders.

Women in Helgesen's study were very concerned about being involved in the work of the organization, keeping relationships healthy and productive, making time for activities that were not directly related to their work (e.g., parenting responsibilities), and maintaining a "big picture" orientation. They also viewed their jobs as only one element of who they were, not as the factor that defined who they were, and they preferred to see themselves at the center of things rather than at the top.

As a result of these values, perspectives, and preferences, women tended to create management structures that were more web-like than hierarchical. Such structures allow more interaction among members of the group, more participation of all players in goal setting and decision making, and greater inclusion.

Helgesen views these differences in the ways women lead as great strengths, strengths that will continue to have dramatic effects on the nature of our organizations. The book provides a provocative analysis of women leaders and the ways in which they can use their different perspectives and values to change organizations.

Joel Barker's leadershift: Five lessons for leaders in the 21st century. 1999. A Star Thrower film. Produced by AMI, St. Paul, MN.

This excellent video features Joel Barker, a futurist. Barker discusses how leaders build bridges between today and tomorrow, and he asserts that the most important role of a leader is to find, recognize, and secure the future.

Barker notes that the foundations to "building bridges" include trust, communication and confidence, all qualities of leaders as described by other experts. Armed with these qualities, leaders can and must exist at all levels and in all endeavors, according to Barker, and he asserts that leadership is no longer about privilege; instead, it is about responsibility.

Through a dynamic video that captures the attention of the viewer, Barker talks about the need for new paradigms, which drive fundamental change in our organizations and society. He offers the following five "lessons" for the 21st century, all of which are wise words of counsel for anyone assuming a leadership role in the coming years.

- ◆ Focus the majority of your efforts on the future.

- ◆ Understand the nature of fundamental change.

- ◆ Appreciate complex systems and how they work.

- ◆ Examine your leadership style to see how it affects productivity.

♦   Create shared vision to build bridges to the future.

This video (Accompanied by a Power Point Presentation on a CD-ROM, a participant workbook, and a facilitator's guide) is an excellent resource that can help us understand that we must dramatically alter our ways of thinking and behaving if we are to make necessary changes and provide much-needed leadership.

Kelly, R.E. 1992. *The power of followership: How to create leaders people want to follow and followers who lead themselves.* New York; Doubleday Currency

Rober Kelley presents one of the best discussions of followership that is available in the literature. His goal in writing this book is to "shift the spotlight toward followership as the important phenomenon to study if we are to understand why organizations succeed or fail" (p. 5), and he achieves that goal extremely well.

The author talks about the increasing emphasis on teams and collaboration and the kind of power that followers can and do have in groups and organizations. He notes that "followers determine not only if someone will be accepted as a leader but also if that leader will be effective" (p. 13) and asserts that effective followers are critical to success.

The term "effective Follower" is not taken lightly in this book. Indeed, Kelley describes five different followership styles, one of which is effective: passive, conformist, pragmatist, alienated, and exemplary. He offers ways to help readers identify their followership styles, argues for the importance of developing one's followership skill, and offers very convincing arguments for why we shold become followers.

This book, therefore, is unique in its attention to a critical but frequently ignored role in the leadership process. It is one that must be read to gain a better appreciation of the concept of followership.

Kouzes, J., and B. Posner. 1987. *The leadership challenge: how to get extraordinary things done in organizations.* San Francisco: Jossey-Bass

This excellent book reflects the author's observations of what leaders do to encourage extraordinary accomplishments when they are leading, not managing. Their classic "five sets of behavioral practices" and "10 behavioral commitments" are described fully, and the importance of leaders having perseverance, having direction, empowering others, being role models, and recognizing others' contributions are all discussed thoroughly.

The book points out that leadership is a skill that can be developed by coaching and through experimental learning. The necessity of purposefully developing one's leadership is advanced, as is the notion that leadership is more important today than ever before if we are to achieve success in the future. The author's remind us that leadership is everyone's business and that everyone should therefor accept the leadership "challenge" on a daily basis.

Kouzes, J. M., and B. Z. Posner. 1993. *Credibility: How leaders gain and lost it... Why people demand it.* **San Francisco: Jossey-Bass.**

The purpose of this book is to explore, in depth, credibility — the quality present in leaders whom constituents (i.e., followers) want to follow. On the basis of extensive research, the authors concluded that people have very high expectations of their leaders and want them to "hold to an ethic of service, [be] genuinely respectful of the intelligence and contributions of their constituents, [and] put principles ahead of politics and other people before self-interests" (p. xvii).

Kouzes and Posner view leadership as a relationship and a service, with credibility clearly at its foundation. This book examines the concept of leadership as a relationship, talks about the benefits of credibility, and discusses the behaviors that convey and establish credibility. Among those behaviors are the following: knowing yourself and your values, appreciating the strengths and talents in your followers, reinforcing shared values, helping others develop to reach their fullest potential, making meaning out of the work or tasks to be done, and sustaining hope in the followers. Ways in which leaders develop, gain, and lose credibility are also discussed.

This analysis stimulates the reader to thoughtfully reflect on her/his own actions and how they establish or undermine credibility. Although other writers imply the significance of credibility in the leader/follower relationship, this book is a valuable contribution to our understanding of how leaders can be most effective. Any discussion of leadership would be incomplete without a discussion of credibility; this book, therefore, is an excellent resource for enhancing such understanding.

Leadership in nursing. 1994. *Holistic Nursing Practice* **9.**

This journal issue offers a thoughtful collection of articles about the nature of leadership, particularly as it relates to nursing. The articles, each of which can be read independently of the others, focus on many significant areas that facilitate an understanding of the complex nature of leadership. Included among those areas are the following: the nature of leadership and ways to conceptualize it that make sense for 21st-century practice; the holistic nature of leadership; transformational leadership, particularly as it relates to women leaders; the significance of followers; ethical aspects of leadership; the preparation of leaders; an exploration of the leadership that is needed to shape a preferred future for nursing; and an analysis of 10 years of research in nursing leadership.

All of the articles in this issue are intended to "provide new insights and to explore important issues related to leadership" (p. vi). They accomplish that goal in a stimulating way that has relevance for our profession.

McCall, M. W. 1998. *High flyers: Developing the next generation of leaders.* **Boston: Harvard Business School Press.**

This book emphasizes corporate executives, with a "bent" that is more toward management than leadership. Despite this, however, McCall presents many interesting ideas about leaders and what needs to be done to prepare individuals to be effective in leadership roles.

The author asserts that "organizations not only overlook people with the potential to develop but also frequently and unintentionally derail the talented people they have identified as high flyers by rewarding them for their flaws, teaching them to behave in ineffective ways, reinforcing narrow perspectives and skills, and inflating their egos" (p. xi). He notes that we often keep people from developing their full potential as leaders. As a result, neither they nor their organizations progress as much as they otherwise could.

McCall firmly believes that leadership can be learned and points out that "the development of leaders is itself a leadership responsibility" (p. xii). Learning leadership, he says, is a "lifelong journey, with its lessons taught by the journey itself" (p. 17). He challenges each of us — as aspiring leaders who must take responsibility for our own growth and as practicing leaders who must take responsibility for the leadership development of others — to attend to the conscious development of ourselves and others as leaders.

McFarland, L., L. Senn, and J. Childress. 1994. *21ˢᵗ century leadership: Dialogues with 100 top leaders.* **New York: The Leadership Press.**

This book is the result of a collaboration among members of two associations — Leadership into the Next Century and the Senn-Delaney Leadership Consulting Group — who set out to identify the foremost thinking about leadership for the 21ˢᵗ century. The authors interviewed 100 of the most prominent leaders of the world (individuals from business, government, education, and other key sectors of society) and asked them for recommendations and ideas on how individuals and organizations could make their visions become realities in the new millennium.

The dialogues consist of numerous ideas on how to be a successful risk taker, how to welcome change, why it is important to be flexible and adaptable, and how to create a vision and succeed. They also encompass the importance of being globally aware, involved in networking, and connected to information of every conceivable type.

After reading this book, one realizes that it is impossible to strategically plan every step of one's professional or personal life. What is important and possible, however, is becoming a part of the dynamic change by forming partnerships with others and continuously reaching for new growth.

Nanus, B. 1992. *Visionary leadership: Creating a compelling sense of direction for your organization.* **San Francisco: Jossey-Bass.**

This is an excellent book about the concept of vision and its importance in the leadership process. Nanus asserts that vision is the key to leadership and that without it, an individual cannot be considered a leader and significant progress cannot be made in our organizations, professions, or societies.

A leader, Nanus explains, must be attuned to the external environment (perhaps more so than the internal one) and be focused on the future, not merely on the present. This kind of direction setting is what vision is all about, and it is what "attracts commitment and energizes people" (p. 16). Vision also serves to create meaning in the lives of the followers and to establish a standard of excellence that applies to everyone.

Nanus also helps the reader understand what vision is not. It is not, he says, prophesy, a mission, factual, true or false, static, or a constraint on actions. Instead, it is a view of the future that arises from one's values, passions, dreams, hopes, and desires to create a better world (or piece of the world).

Nanus offers many realistic and helpful strategies with which leaders can develop a compelling vision for the future of their organizations or groups. He also helps the reader think about ways to implement these strategies.

Porter-O'Grady, T., and C. Wilson. 1995. *The leadership revolution in health care: Altering systems, changing behaviors.* **Gaithersburg, MD: Aspen Publications.**

The primary theme throughout this book is that healthcare providers must measure and track indicators of quality and that nurses, in particular, must be clinically skilled as well as proficient in business. Outcome management must be a significant focus of nursing, so that the impact of nursing interventions on patient care and patient health status can be documented.

The authors point out the significance of changing our beliefs about functioning under "orders from the top" and suggest that nurses need to get involved now in the leadership revolution that is occurring in healthcare. O'Grady and Wilson note that it is no longer acceptable for nurses merely to be responsible. They must also be accountable for helping to attain a proper balance among access to, quality of, and costs associated with *healthcare* delivery, not just *nursing care* delivery. The authors assert that all providers of care must form partnerships with patients and managers to provide the highest quality care possible.

In addition to these thoughtful and sometimes unsettling challenges, this comprehensive book also offers a wide array of resources that help the reader better understand leadership and themselves as leaders. Appendices include a leadership survey, sample leadership training activities, guidelines for leadership development, and an example of a vision and mission statement.

Rosenbach, W.E., and R.L. Taylor, eds. (1998). *Contemporary issues in leadership.* **4ᵗʰ ed. Boulder, CO: Westview Press.**

This book (and all previous editions) is one of the best collections of readings about leadership. None of the articles — many of which have been published originally elsewhere and several of which are classics in the field — has to date focused specifically on nursing, but each of them offers many rich ideas that could easily be applied to a nursing context. The book, therefore, is valuable to students and teachers of nursing.

The editors drawing on experts in each area and include articles from journals like *Harvard Business Review, Journal of Leadership Studies,* and the *Journal of Creative Behavior*. Because of this, the book is exciting and includes diverse perspectives. Although several of the articles are taken from management journals, they are clearly focused on leadership. This collection is so valuable in part because it does not confuse management and leadership.

Note: All previous editions of this book also are valuable and include collections of different readings. The publication dates of those editions are as follows: 1ˢᵗ edition, early 1980s; 2ⁿᵈ edition, 1989; 3ʳᵈ edition, 1993.

Sinetar, M. 1998. *The mentor's spirit: Life lessons on leadership and the art of encouragement.* **New York: St. Martin's Press.**

This book is another excellent publication by the best-selling author of *Do What You Love... The Money Will Follow* and *To Build the Life You Want, Create the Work You Love: The Spiritual Dimension of Entrepreneuring.* It discusses the art of encouragement, which is the word Sinetar uses to mean mentoring. She describes 12 lessons of mentoring and explains how one can be mentored and how one can mentor others. Realistic strategies and easy-to-follow plans for the mentor and protégé are discussed.

This essential book is easy to read, and it encourages the reader to become involved in a mentor relationship. Sinetar's main point, which echoes throughout the book, is that no matter what one might think, a single person is not the center of the world — it really is worthwhile to reach out to, network with, encourage, and mentor others.

Staub, R. E. 1996. *The heart of leadership.* **Provo, UT: Executive Excellence Publishing.**

This comprehensive book provides step-by-step advice on how to develop effective leadership skills, as well as skills for becoming a productive follower. The author advocates the following 12 practices of leadership: providing guidance through shared vision, focusing on purpose, creating followership, setting standards while eliciting goals, reading and understanding others, providing resources, liberating motivation, supporting others, providing feedback, practicing principled flexibility, soliciting personal feedback, and cultivating the heart of courage.

Staub is a strong believer in everyone working together to lead an organization or group, not just one or two leaders "at the top." Reading this book reaffirms the notion, expressed by so many other experts on leadership, that true leadership is possible for people who can master their attitudes, express their ideas, and act on their dreams.

Vance, C. 1979. Women leaders: Modern day heroines or social deviants? *Image* **11:37–41.**

Although it is more than 20 years old, this article is worth reading. It talks about how women who provide leadership are often seen as social deviants, as individuals who fail to follow the norms of society, who fail to "stay in their place," and who seem to want to take on male roles. Because such ideas can still be found in our organizations today, the notion of "deviant" is still relevant.

Vance's discussion of how risk taking and genuine leadership can be viewed negatively alerts the reader of the need for personal strength, clarity of vision, and commitment in those who will be leaders. Although some may see leaders as heroines, others see them as power-hungry people who want to control others and create their own world. Thus, would-be leaders must be prepared to take on the challenge, find ways to develop collaborative relationships with followers, and persevere in pursuing their visions and turning them into reality.

Vance, C. and R. K. Olson. 1998. *The mentor connection in nursing.* **New York: Springer.**

This book is not presented as a "leadership" book, but the nature of its focus — mentoring — makes it quite relevant to any study of leadership and followership. In addition, the book itself is one strategy used by these authors to realize their own vision of nurses mentoring each other. Its roots were in the 1977 and 1984 doctoral dissertations of the two authors, and it crystallized over more than a decade of collaboration.

Mentoring, these authors say, is a unique type of developmental relationship. It involves colleagues helping each other grow and learn, it empowers each person in the relationship, and it is a means to "strengthen the profession by ensuring an adequate supply of competent practitioners and leaders" (p. 3). As such, mentoring must become a natural part of the practice of all nurses.

Through the use of personal "stories," many of nursing's accomplished leaders help the reader understand the nature of mentoring, the value of such relationships, and the relevance of mentoring to nursing. Various contributing authors talk about negotiating the mentor relationship, peer mentoring, the privilege and responsibility of mentoring, mentoring in the practice and the academic setting, and global and cross-cultural mentoring. Many of these discussions incorporate personal experiences and are therefore particularly moving, meaningful, and memorable.

This is an excellent resource for understanding the phenomenon of mentoring. It is also a valuable collection of personal stories that present a positive view of our profession and that serve as "anchors" for neophytes who are looking for or hoping for a mentoring relationship. It is, in essence, an informative, inspiring book.

Wheatley, M. 1994. *Leadership and the new science: Learning about organization from an orderly universe.* **San Francisco: Berrett-Koehler Publishers.**

This is Wheatley's seminal work on the New Science. Contrary to the Scientific or Newtonian Model, which centered around step-by-step planning, the New Science emphasizes the importance of exploring and accepting things the way they occur, as viewed from the perspectives of quantum physics, chaos theory, and biology.

Wheatley discusses how leaders and those responsible for running organizations can benefit from application of the New Science. She asserts that by moving toward holism and appreciating the intricate relationships that exist between and among all things, one can develop and effectively use methods to change how people act, how they work, and how they view life. As a result of this interconnectedness between every single thing in the world (actually everything *plus* the world, according to Wheatley), every moment of one's day is dynamic and unpredictable.

Wheatley explains how order and chaos can be seen as identical images and how these two seemingly opposite forces actually drive each other. Using natural phenomena (such as the evolution of the Grand Canyon, a babbling brook, and stormy weather), Wheatley creates complexity from simplicity and excites the reader with ideas of how the future will evolve from the whole rather than from its parts. This is a "must-read" book for anyone interested in learning more about chaos theory and the New Science.

Wheatley, M., and M. Kellner-Rogers. 1996. *A simpler way.* **San Francisco: Berrett-Koehler Publishers.**

This book offers a way of thinking about life in a dynamic and totally different way. It is critical reading for those who wish to better understanding the New Science of Leadership. The authors share a magnificent collection of photographs of life, poems that convey the importance of being oneself, and narratives about simpler ways of viewing what most people define as a stress-filled, nonenjoyable life.

This is a remarkable book about how to view life within the vastness of the universe. The authors discuss how life "self-organizes" without our planning every minute of every day and how this organization creates our identities. The advantages of seeing the world self-organize without human manipulation is challenged and discussed, and ways to foster more creativity, freedom, and "real" meaning in life are generated. In addition, the notions of play, organization, self, emergence, and coherence are explored.

Zaleznik, A. 1977. Managers and leaders: Are they different? *Harvard Business Review* **55:67–78.**

This article is essential reading. It is one of the earliest works in which leadership is clearly distinguished from management; as such, it is a classic in the field. Zaleznik talks about the differences between managers and leaders in terms of how they relate to other people, to the organization, and to goals. He explores different conceptions of work, different perspectives on solitary activity, and different views about conflict and status quo held by leaders and managers. For purposes of illustration, the author talks about leaders and managers in the extreme, but he does acknowledge that managers can also be leaders and leaders also can be managers. This article is clearly written and is extremely helpful in clarifying the distinctions between these two related phenomena. It is required reading in the quest to understand leadership.

Appendix D

Ideas for Student Leadership Projects

IDEAS FOR STUDENT LEADERSHIP PROJECTS

1. Submit a manuscript to a nursing journal on a topic such as the following: your role in volunteering at a homeless shelter; the need to develop healthcare policies to ensure that people with tuberculosis have proper medical treatment; or your experiences working with a legislator in town, city, or state government.

2. "Shadow" a leader in an organization of your choice for 6 days, approximately 5 hours per day. Develop personal objectives for your experience related to your growth in at least five areas of leadership (e.g., vision clarification, team building, communication skills, collaboration and networking, facilitating change, etc.).

3. Collect data from people experiencing a health problem that is of particular interest to you. Assimilate the information you gather with what you find in the literature and present it to an agency that may be able to assist you in solving or managing the health problem. Collaborate with individuals from that agency to write a grant in support of a program that would help the population of concern and address the identified health problem.

4. As a member of a School of Nursing committee, participate in solving a student-related problem, developing a new policy, creating a new program or initiative, evaluating program outcome data, or writing a newsletter. Be actively involved with the chair of the committee. Negotiate to co-chair one of the subcommittees with a faculty member.

5. Select a topic with which you were involved in a previous course (e.g., nursing research, community health, care of chronically ill children, etc.), and work on the topic/project in a broader scope or with narrower, intensive focus.

6. Collaborate with staff of your university's healthcare center to develop a program that would improve student/staff communication, widen the scope of care, offer a new type of care, or develop new policies on healthcare issues that are particularly relevant to college students.

7. Become involved in your university's nursing laboratory or library in order to improve access, enhance student compliance regarding use of the resources, and develop an evaluation method for garnering increased student input to the services offered in the laboratory or library.

8. Develop a critical path, evidence-based protocol, committee, or a brochure or poster for teaching patients that can be used in one of the units in which you have had a clinical experience.